YOUR COMPLETE GUIDE TO

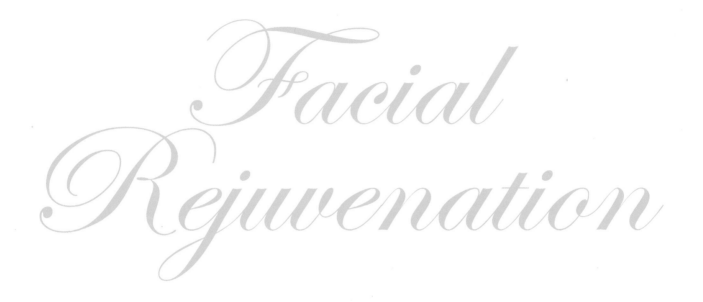

Facial Rejuvenation

William Truswell, M.D. • Neil A. Gordon, M.D.

Jon Mendelsohn, M.D. • David A.F. Ellis, M.D.

Harrison C. Putman III, M.D.

Addicus Books
Omaha, Nebraska

An Addicus Nonfiction Book

ISBN 10: 1-886039-20-8
          13: 978-1-886039-20-9

Cover design by Peri Poloni-Gabriel
Illustrations by Jack Kusler
Typography by Darcy Lijoodi

This book is not intended to serve as a substitute for a physician.
Nor is it the authors' intent to give medical advice contrary to that of an attending physician.

Library of Congress Cataloging-in-Publication Data
Your complete guide to facial rejuvenation / William Truswell ... [et al.].
   p. cm.
   Includes index.
   ISBN-10: 1-886039-20-8 (alk. paper)
   ISBN-13: 978-1-886039-20-9 (alk. paper)
1. Facelift--Popular works. I. Truswell, William, 1946-

RD119.5.F33Y68 2006
617.5'20592--dc22   2006017381

Addicus Books, Inc.
P.O. Box 45327
Omaha, Nebraska 68145
www.AddicusBooks.com

Printed in the United States of America
10 9 8 7 6 5 4 3 2 1

Contents

Acknowledgments

My gratitude goes to those people whose patience and support ease me through my day: my wife, Lynn, who manages my practice and is an individual of great intelligence and forbearance, and my children, Jason and Jody, of whom I am so proud.

I also express my thanks to the wonderful women who work with me, my nurses Kathy, Lisa, and Cozette; my surgical assistant, Laura; my patient coordinator, Jessica; my skin care technicians, Johanne and Nancy; and my business staff, Nancy and Darci. These are the individuals to whom I dedicate this book. I also wish to acknowledge the American Academy of Facial Plastic and Reconstructive Surgery—the resource for education, guidance, support, and fraternity for facial plastic surgeons throughout the world.

—*William Truswell, M.D.*

I would like to thank my family for all of their love, support, and encouragement over the years. I would like to especially thank my wonderful and inspirational grandmother, Sally; my Mom and Dad for their unconditional love; Susie for her encouragement; and Mark and Scott for their support and kindness. I am especially grateful for the love and the joy that I receive daily from my twins, Hannah and Benny, as they inspire me to be the best I can every moment.

I would also like to extend my sincere thanks and gratitude to my outstanding team at Advanced Cosmetic Surgery & Laser Center. Their dedication to our vision and our patients is superb, and I appreciate their tireless efforts. Thank you.

Finally, I wish to thank all the patients whom I have been fortunate enough to care for. Every day I derive tremendous satisfaction in the work I do and from the relationships I have developed with you. I am hopeful that this will last a lifetime.

— *Jon Mendelsohn, M.D.*

For their love, support, and patience throughout this endeavor and throughout my professional career, I would like to acknowledge these special people in my life: my wonderful wife, Mary, and our children, Michelle and Christopher. Mary, you have been my life partner inside and out of the operating room. You have contributed immeasurably to my professional development as a surgeon and my personal development as a husband and father. Michelle and Chris, I take great pride in the fine human beings you have become and in your considerable accomplishments in your young lives.

Thank you to my superlative staff, Debbie, Mary, Kara, and Mary, for your loyalty, devotion, patience, and hard work in sharing my vision for our practice.

Acknowledgment is also due to the American Academy of Facial Plastic and Reconstructive Surgery, a truly remarkable organization for its excellence in leadership, education, fellowship, and social responsibility throughout the years.

—*Harrison C. Putman III, M.D.*

I would first like to thank my wife, Stephanie, whose love, support, and encouragement have allowed me to successfully pursue my personal and professional goals. She is my personal counterbalance and life confidant. I am especially blessed to have two wonderful daughters, Rachel and Lia, who give me joy and pleasure on a daily basis and give my life a sense of purpose. I would also like to thank my parents, Sandi and George, for their unconditional love and support.

I wish to express my thanks to my entire staff at The Retreat at Split Rock, New England Surgical Center and Split Rock Surgery Associates. Their drive and commitment to excellence has allowed our vision of facial plastic surgery to be accomplished and they devote themselves daily to the diverse and complex tasks necessary to consistently achieve our goals.

Finally, I would like to acknowledge the American Academy of Facial Plastic and Reconstructive Surgery for the education, support, and commitment to the field and profession of facial plastic surgery. I would not be the person and professional I am today if not for all the people mentioned above.

—*Neil A. Gordon, M.D.*

I would like to thank my wife, Craig, for her love and support. She and our children, Whitney and Trevor, have always been enthusiastic supporters of my endeavors, allowing me to pursue the goals I set for myself many years ago.

Thank you to Barb, my practice manager, who has been instrumental in keeping me organized and the office running smoothly. My other right hand, Helen, who is my skin care specialist and patient coordinator, offers exceptional enthusiasm, energy, and knowledge. Barb, Helen, and my nurse, Karen, have been the building blocks of my practice.

For the last twenty years I have had a fellowship in facial plastic surgery sponsored both by the University of Toronto and the American Academy of Facial Plastic and Reconstructive Surgery. The benefits are twofold. Not only can I teach surgeons the craft of facial plastic surgery, but I also learn from them. Thank you to all my fellows who have participated in my practice. They have gone on to enhance the proficiency of facial plastic surgery and impart their knowledge to others.

I would also like to thank the American Academy of Facial Plastic and Reconstructive Surgery, for its education, support, and guidance for facial plastic surgeons both in North America and internationally. I am proud to be a member of such an organization.

—*David Ellis, M.D.*

Introduction

*D*o you feel younger than you look? If so, you are one among many who feel this way. Many of us take good care of ourselves—we exercise and eat right. Yet, we look in the mirror and see a reflection that doesn't match our inner self. This is, no doubt, one of the reasons why more and more Americans are choosing to undergo cosmetic surgery: They want to look as good as they feel.

If you are considering a facelift, this book will help you better understand your options. There are various types of facelifts and we will explain each of them, their benefits, and how they are performed. With improved technology and refined techniques, these surgeries are safer and more effective than ever. Nevertheless, there are side effects and risks to any surgical procedure, even minimally invasive ones. We will explain what they are and how to minimize them. Also, you will see before-and-after photos that will show you the results of the procedures on other patients.

You will learn why your face ages and what you can do to combat that aging. In addition, you will be provided information to help you locate qualified facial plastic surgeons. You will also learn what questions to ask them to learn more about a specific procedure and determine whether the procedure, as well as the doctor, is right for you. We hope you'll find this book helpful.

CHAPTER ONE

A Change of Face: How We Age

1

A Change of Face: How We Age

When you look into a mirror, do you like what you see?

If you don't, give yourself an "instant facelift." Place your fingers beneath your jaw or at the hairline and give your face a gentle tug. For a moment, your younger self will peer back at you. Frown lines will be smoothed away, crow's-feet will have taken flight, and your cheeks will look higher and firmer.

What happens when you release your fingers? Do you see the effects of gravity—some sag in the skin, some wrinkles, or folds, a bit of a tired look? The corners of your mouth may have turned down, eliminating your former natural, youthful smile. The years may have etched lines on your face, making you look older than you actually feel.

Don't despair. Like thousands of individuals who have experienced the same feelings, you may be able to reclaim your younger beauty by seeking facial rejuvenation. Every year more than 100,000 people, 85 percent of them women, choose to have facelifts and other techniques to counter the effects of aging. If the instant facelift made you look and feel younger even momentarily, then you, too, may want to consider a facelift.

Signs of Facial Aging

Eyelids

The eyelids are often the first harbingers of aging. Extra skin in upper and lower lids and bagginess under the eyes may become noticeable. We start to notice wrinkles, crow's-feet, at the corners of the eyes. We will also see wrinkles starting to develop across the forehead and between the eyes.

The area just below the lower lid may become discolored, turning a light gray, green, or brown. In very fair-skinned people, the thinning skin's transparency reveals vascular and muscle tissue beneath. This coloration isn't fixed by surgery, but it can be disguised with cosmetics.

Cheeks and Midface

Some of the earliest signs of aging occur in the midface region when the *malar fat pads*—the pads of fat that cover our cheekbones—begin to slide downward. When we are young, these fat pads sit on the upper cheekbones, creating a fullness to the cheeks and the regions under the eyes. However, as these pads begin to sag with age, they produce a number of changes in the face. We notice a hollowing under the eyes and in the upper cheeks; the nasolabial folds deepen (these are the creases that run from each side of the nose to the corners of the mouth); and the corners of the mouth start to turn downward. These changes typically create a tired look.

Jawline

As we get older, the skin and soft tissue along the jawline sags, becoming loose and thin. Sooner or later we develop jowls, excess fat and skin below the jawline, which "washes" away the middle third of the jawline.

Neck

As we age, loose skin droops between the thin muscles, the *platysma* muscles, of the neck. These muscles also droop with the skin, often appearing as bands or chords of loose skin. These bands are masked by fat in individuals with heavy necks.

Surface Changes in Skin

The outermost layer of our skin, composed of dead cells, is called the *stratum corneum*. As we age, the composition of this layer of surface skin changes. In our teens and twenties, every time we wash, this outermost layer comes off, leaving a fresh new surface. However, around age thirty, the stratum corneum becomes "sticky" and those dead cells begin to adhere. Pores open wider and look larger; wrinkles and discolorations appear. The skin dries and becomes thinner. Facial skin loses its youthful, translucent depth and glow and takes on a flat, matted look.

"With the advancements in surgical techniques, safe anesthesia, and minimally invasive procedures, I find a facelift procedure is a much less daunting prospect for most patients now than in the past."

—Harrison C. Putman III, M.D.

Why Your Face Ages

There are extrinsic and intrinsic reasons why skin ages, and the distinction between them is important. The intrinsic causes relate to gravity and your genes, things that cannot be controlled. The extrinsic causes, which *can* be controlled, include such things as sun exposure, tobacco use, weight fluctuations, stress, chronic illness, exposure to harsh climates, alcohol consumption, and poor nutrition.

What You Can't Change

Genes

The rate at which our skin and soft tissue ages is affected by our genes. You've probably noticed some people seem to have fewer wrinkles and firmer-looking skin than other people their age. This may be partly due to their genetics. Sometimes an entire family will retain an unusually youthful appearance. In other cases, the "family face" might keep pace right along with the calendar.

Cell Breakdown

As we grow older, connective tissues in the dermis, a layer of tissues below the skin, begin to break down, and cells aren't able to repair themselves as quickly as they did when we were younger. The connections between our bone structure and the soft tissue loosen and cause the facial tissue to droop. The production of both *collagen*, the main protein of skin tissue, and *elastin*, a stretchable protein, diminishes. As collagen production diminishes, our skin begins to droop and wrinkle.

There are two types of wrinkles. *Static* wrinkles are visible when the face is at rest. *Dynamic* wrinkles are those we see only when the face moves, such as smile lines that aren't deeply carved. We also lose muscle volume and tone as we age, which contributes to sagging.

What You Can Change

Exposure to Sun

Excessive sun exposure is the number one cause of premature aging. Early wrinkling and "age spots," known as *photoaging* and *solar lentigos*, are signs that skin has not been adequately protected from the sun. You can't undo damage that occurred in your younger years, but you can start now to protect your skin from further damage by the regular use of sunscreen and other protection from the sun's UVA rays. These rays penetrate most deeply and are most closely associated with premature aging.

Every day, year-round, apply full-spectrum sunscreen (SPF 15 or higher), and avoid exposure during the midday hours when the sun's rays reach Earth most directly. For about ten minutes a day, however, do let sunlight reach unprotected skin, because sun on skin triggers the body's production of vitamin D, which is crucial for bone growth.

Remember that, in addition to the sun, harsh weather such as wind and cold can also age skin that is not well protected and regularly moisturized.

Smoking

Smoking is harmful to every organ in your body, including your skin—the body's largest organ. Smoking causes lung cancer, heart disease, and other ailments. It also decreases the flow of blood and oxygen to your entire body, including your facial skin, thus starving your skin of nutrients. For this reason, most smokers appear to age more rapidly than nonsmokers. Smoking also produces fine wrinkles in the upper lip.

Yo-Yo Diets

Repeatedly losing and gaining weight isn't just hard on you emotionally, but repeated stretching of the skin as your body changes from heavy to slim to heavy to slim contributes to facial sagging over time.

Stress

No one can prevent all stress—it is a part of life—but limiting it, learning to relax, and living at a saner pace can influence the rate of cell aging. The stresses of chronic, stress-induced illness will leave their mark on the skin's appearance, too, so it's important to choose and maintain a balanced lifestyle. Staying as healthy as possible helps your face look younger.

Alcohol Consumption

Excessive use of alcohol dehydrates and ravages the skin, leaving it pasty and sallow. When you abuse alcohol, you tend to be undernourished, making your skin and hair dry

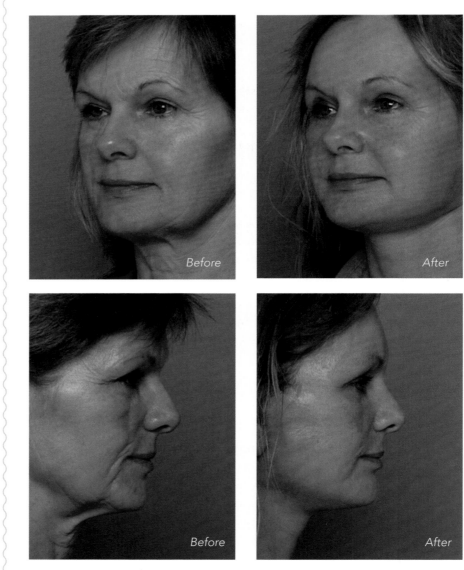

To maximize the effects of facial cosmetic surgery, your surgeon may recommend other procedures to complement a facelift. The woman above had a brow lift along with a facelift.

and causing cracked lips; alcohol abuse can also aggravate acne and can make your skin look puffy.

Poor Nutrition

A wholesome diet helps cells renew themselves. Plenty of antioxidant-rich fruits and vegetables, whole grains, lean proteins, and healthful monounsaturated fats such as olive oil nourish your skin along with the rest of your body. A diet heavy in sugar, saturated fat, and junk food will do just the opposite. A low-quality diet shows on your face and speeds its aging.

Dehydration

Your skin needs lots of water. Water plumps up cells and helps to flush toxins from the body. Drinking eight glasses of water a day will allow your cells to work more efficiently, and your skin will show it.

How Can Cosmetic Surgery Help?

Cosmetic surgery, such as a facelift, can reverse many of the signs of aging. The intent of any cosmetic surgery is not to achieve perfection, but rather improvement. The first step toward having a cosmetic surgery procedure is finding the right cosmetic surgeon.

"The greater the degree of facial aging, the greater the need is to address both the upper and lower portions of the face. It's important to achieve balance when rejuvenating the face."
—Neil A. Gordon, M.D.

CHAPTER TWO

Choosing a Cosmetic Surgeon

2

Choosing a Cosmetic Surgeon

You've made the decision. You want to rejuvenate your face. Now the question is, "How do I find the best surgeon to perform the procedure?" Perhaps you already know the right cosmetic surgeon for the job. If not, finding the right surgeon is an important decision that merits your time and effort. You want a skilled facial plastic surgeon who has a solid reputation. And equally important, you want a doctor you "click" with—one you trust and feel comfortable with.

You might meet with only one surgeon and choose him or her to perform your facelift. Or you might choose to meet with two or three and then determine which surgeon will be best for you. Either way, meeting face-to-face will help you decide.

Ways to Find a Cosmetic Surgeon

If you flip open the yellow pages or do an online search, you'll find a number of cosmetic surgeons. Across the nation, there are several thousand cosmetic surgeons; perhaps many of them practice in your area. How do you find the right one?

Word of Mouth

Even in today's world of high technology, one of the best ways to find a qualified surgeon is still through the old-fashioned word of mouth. When patients are satisfied with their experience and their results, they often become a doctor's best source of advertising. If you have friends or relatives who have had facial plastic surgery, ask them about their experience and who performed their surgery. Ask them to describe their relationship with the surgeon. What level of confidence did they have in their surgeon? Ask about the expectations they had going in, and whether those expectations were met.

Furthermore, ask about the staff and the office suite. Did all these factors add up to a pleasing experience? How did the physician relate to the patient? Is the surgeon someone in whom you could place your trust?

Referrals from Other Professionals

Your primary care physician or other physicians, such as your gynecologist or dermatologist, likely have patients who have had cosmetic surgery. Ask these doctors for a referral to a surgeon whom they know and respect. Local hospitals and your local county medical society may also be able to refer you to competent facial plastic surgeons.

Non-health professionals may also be a source for referrals. Hair dressers and spa facialists often have customers who have had cosmetic surgery procedures and who can recommend good facial plastic surgeons.

Online Searches

The Internet has made it easy to search for virtually any kind of information, including information about cosmetic surgeons. Some of the best Web sites to visit are those of the professional associations of cosmetic surgeons. Members in these societies are accepted by their peers and have to maintain continuing medical education in their specialty. Each of these organizations has an online "physician finder" function to help you find a qualified expert near you. These organizations include:

- American Academy of Facial Plastic and Reconstructive Surgery
  www.facemd.org

- American Society for Aesthetic Plastic Surgery
  www.surgery.org

- American Society of Plastic Surgeons
  www.plasticsurgery.org

You'll also find the Web sites of various cosmetic surgeons. Be sure to do your research and carefully check the credentials of any surgeon you find online.

"It is important to have confidence and trust in the facial plastic surgeon one chooses. This includes his/her competence and experience, but also honesty about goals, the process, and results that can be achieved."
—Jon Mendelsohn, M.D.

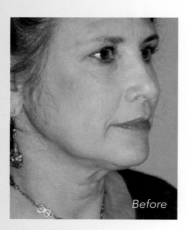

Before

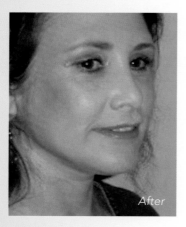

After

Facelift

Qualifications of a Cosmetic Surgeon

Certainly you want a surgeon who has the proper qualifications. But what qualifications should you look for? When searching for a surgeon for your facial rejuvenation procedure, you need to look for several things. The surgeon should be a licensed physician with adequate training, board certification, and sufficient experience performing facial rejuvenation procedures.

Training and Education

Becoming a facial plastic surgeon requires the completion of several years of formal education and training. Education requirements include graduating from a four-year college or university with a bachelor's degree and then graduating from a four-year accredited medical school with an M.D. degree. An accredited medical school is one that meets national standards set by a national authority for medical education programs. Doctors who wish to perform facial plastic surgery must then complete at least five years of additional hospital training called a residency. During a residency, the physician in training, known as a resident, works closely with senior-level surgeons to observe their work and gain hands-on experience in the operating room. Once the residency is completed, the doctor can go into practice as a facial plastic surgeon. Or, he or she may choose to apply for additional training in an accredited fellowship. A fellowship is a program in which the surgeon specializes in advanced techniques and patient care in facial plastic surgery.

Once all formal training in complete, facial plastic surgeons are required to take continuing education courses throughout their careers.

Licensure

In order to practice medicine, a facial plastic surgeon is required to be licensed by the state in which the surgeon's office is located. State licensing is mandatory, and licenses are usually granted only to medical school graduates who pass a comprehensive exam. Each state has slightly different requirements, so if a physician relocates, he or she needs to acquire a new state license. To verify that your facial plastic surgeon is licensed, you can check with your state's medical board. You can also check with the medical board to see if any complaints have been lodged or disciplinary actions taken against a surgeon. A list of state medical boards and links to their Web sites are available on the Federation of State Medical Boards Web site (www.fsmb.org/directory_smb.html).

Board Certification

If you've done your research, you've probably heard that it's important to select a "board-certified" facial plastic surgeon. But what does it mean to be board-certified, and why is it important? Board certification means that a facial plastic surgeon has completed an accredited residency program of at least five years and has passed written and oral exams given by either the American Board of Otolaryngology (head and neck surgery) or the American Board of Plastic Surgery. Once a doctor is certified by the board, he or she is called a diplomate. A physician whose certification is pending is called a candidate. You can verify board certification on the American Board of Medical Specialties (ABMS) Web site (www.abms.org).

A physician isn't required to be board-certified to practice cosmetic surgery. In fact, board certification is a completely voluntary process. However, for your safety and peace of mind, you should choose only a cosmetic surgeon who is board-certified. Board certification provides the assurance that your surgeon is adequately trained. Facial plastic surgeons are required to renew their certification every ten years. Be sure your surgeon's certification is up to date.

In addition to board certification, a surgeon can seek additional certification in facial plastic surgery. The American Board of Facial Plastic and Reconstructive Surgery (ABFPRS) offers certification to surgeons who are already board-certified. To qualify for certification from the ABFPRS, a surgeon must complete a two-day comprehensive exam, must have been in practice for at least two years, must have completed at least 100 facial plastic surgeries, and must subscribe to a code of ethics. Choosing a surgeon who is certified by the ABFPRS offers you additional assurance that your surgeon is an experienced facial plastic surgeon. You can verify an American or a Canadian surgeon's certification by the ABFPRS at the organization's Web site (www.abfprs.org).

Experience

We always hear that it is important to choose a surgeon who has experience in performing facial plastic surgery. However, what constitutes experience? Do we consider a surgeon experienced if he or she performs two surgeries a month? Or should it be ten or fifteen surgeries a month? You want a doctor who does facelifts as a regular part of his or her practice, not one who occasionally performs them. Ask the doctor how many facelifts he or

In Canada, cosmetic surgeons are certified by the Royal College of Physicians and Surgeons of Canada (www.royalcollege.ca). Once certified by this organization, the surgeon is considered a Fellow of the Royal College of Physicians and Surgeons of Canada. Canadian surgical centers are accredited by the Canadian Association of Accreditation of Ambulatory Surgery Facilities.

she performs; if it's fewer than two a month, then you might continue to look for a surgeon who has more experience and for whom facelifts represent a more significant portion of his or her work. Generally, the greater the experience, the greater the skill.

Your Consultation

A consultation with the cosmetic surgeon is your opportunity to have a totally candid discussion about your desire to have cosmetic surgery. Don't be shy. Only when you are totally honest can the surgeon tell you what is possible. Explain why you'd like a facelift. Describe what makes you unhappy about your face and how you would like it to look. Be precise about what you want, but also be open to suggestions from the surgeon. You might learn about procedures you didn't know were available, or it's possible that you'll learn that a facelift won't do what you want it to do.

The surgeon will let you know what you can expect from a facelift. He or she will explain how the procedure is performed and how anesthesia will be administered. The surgeon will also discuss possible complications and risks and what to expect after the surgery in terms of recuperating and returning to work.

Medical History

The doctor will collect your medical history, which you should obtain from your primary care physician and take with you (or have sent from your primary care physician). Included in this medical history are these records:

- Past and current medical conditions, including hospitalizations, operations, and any noninvasive cosmetic procedures that you've had done
- Lab work, such as CT scans, MRIs, and X-rays
- Information on allergies to foods, medicines, soaps, and anything else
- Dental history
- Eye exam and eye surgery information
- All medications that you are currently taking, including nonprescription medications and any dietary supplements such as vitamins and herbs

The surgeon will give you instructions that explain which medications and supplements to avoid because of the increased risk of bleeding during surgery. These include aspirin, warfarin (Coumadin), vitamin E, and St. John's Wort, among others. As mentioned earlier, since smoking constricts the blood vessels and can impair healing, the surgeon will recommend that you stop smoking at least two weeks prior to any scheduled surgery. Some surgeons wait until an individual commits to having a procedure before providing these instructions; they then discuss these directives at a pre-op office visit.

Your surgeon will also discuss any conditions, chronic or otherwise, that may make it unwise for you to have facial surgery. These include:

- Uncontrolled high blood pressure
- Blood disorders, such as excessive bleeding or clotting, or a family history of blood disorders
- A history of severe scarring
- Connective tissue disorders
- Chronic heart, lung, liver, or kidney disease
- Long-term steroid use or use of other drugs (such as Accutane for acne)
- Endocrine disorders of the thyroid, parathyroid, or adrenal glands
- Uncontrolled diabetes
- Osteoporosis or other bone disorders
- An autoimmune disease such as lupus or rheumatoid arthritis
- Obesity or anorexia

Physical Examination

The doctor will examine your facial features, skin, bone structure, and expressions. Part of this exam will likely include the physician's taking photos of you. Some surgeons will take a digital photo of you that can be modified on a computer screen to give you an idea what the results of your facelift might look like. This will become your "before" photo, which you'll be able to compare to your "after" photos once your facelift is done.

Seeing Patient Photos

During a consultation, the surgeon should show you a number of before-and-after photos of some of his other facelift patients. These photos should be not only of beautiful people, but also of average-looking people. This will help you gain a realistic perspective on both the doctor's skills and what you might expect from your own facelift.

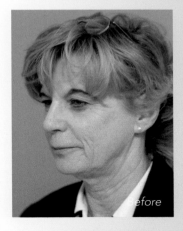

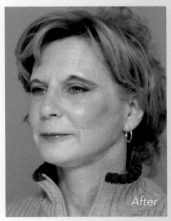

Facelift

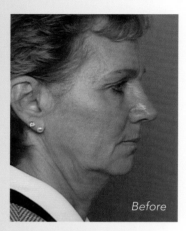
Before

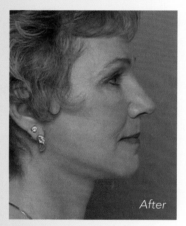
After

Facelift

Also, the office can arrange to give you the phone numbers of former patients who can tell you about their experience with the surgeon. Most surgeons have patients who have agreed to be contacted by phone or in person for such purposes.

Trust and Communication

Listen to your intuition. By the time your consultation is complete, you will likely have a good sense of whether you trust the surgeon. The before-and-after photos might look great, and the surgeon might have impressive credentials, but perhaps he or she seems rushed and doesn't take the time to respond to your questions thoroughly. It's difficult to place trust in a doctor who seems disinterested or too busy for your questions. If, however, the surgeon relates well to you, treats you with respect, and takes the time to educate you on the process, he or she will likely gain your trust. If you have trust in and a good rapport with the surgeon and he or she has the right credentials, experience, and skills, then you may have found your doctor.

Informed Consent

Once you agree to have a surgeon perform your facelift, he or she will have you sign an informed consent form, which states that the procedure and risks have been explained to you. Read the consent form carefully and make sure you understand it before you sign it. If you have any questions, ask your physician.

These forms vary slightly from surgeon to surgeon, but may include the following:

- Authorization for the surgeon to perform the procedure
- Authorization for anesthesia to be administered
- Authorization for the surgeon to perform any additional procedures deemed necessary in case of emergency or to achieve the desired results
- Authorization for the surgeon to take before-and-after photos and/or video
- Acknowledgment that you've been fully informed about your procedure
- Acknowledgment that you've been fully informed about the possible risks involved
- Acknowledgment that there are no guarantees about the results

- Acknowledgment that any computer imaging you were shown isn't a guarantee of the results you'll achieve
- Certification that you have truthfully disclosed all medical conditions, allergies, medications you take, and smoking habits
- Certification that you agree to follow the surgeon's instructions

Financial Considerations

Generally, cosmetic surgery is not covered by insurance. There is often confusion about why insurance will often pay for reconstructive surgery, but not cosmetic surgery. What's the difference between these types of surgeries? Reconstructive surgery is performed to correct abnormalities resulting either from birth defects or injuries. The intent is to make the body normal. Elective cosmetic surgery, on the other hand, involves reshaping normal structures of the body to improve one's appearance and self-esteem.

Most doctors require the entire fee to be paid prior to a cosmetic surgery procedure. There are three types of costs associated with a facelift: surgical fees, facility fees, and anesthesia fees. Surgical fees vary from surgeon to surgeon and from region to region, but in general you can expect to pay from $5,000 to $15,000 for a standard facelift; however, some fees may go as high as $30,000. Surgeon availability is also a factor in determining fees. The costs for the surgical facility will typically be $1,500 to $3,500. If your procedure requires anesthesia, the anesthesia fees will range from about $750 to $3,500. These fees may be set or determined by the length of the operation. Be cautious and questioning of doctors who quote fees that are much lower than those of other surgeons in your region.

When you ask about fees, make sure the fee you are quoted is not the surgical fee alone. You may wish to ask your surgeon if he or she has a financing program available.

The Surgical Center

Facelifts are most often, but not always, performed as outpatient surgery in a surgical suite. Occasionally they are performed in hospitals. If your doctor performs surgery in a surgical suite, ask whether the suite has been accredited. When a facility is accredited, you are assured that its doctors and staff meet nationally recognized health care standards. Accredited centers also have established relationships with local hospitals in case an

$\mathcal{Q}$uestions to ask your surgeon

1. How many facelifts do you perform monthly?

2. Am I a good candidate for a facelift?

3. Are there other treatments that would accomplish what I want?

4. Are my expectations realistic?

5. Will I have postsurgical pain?

6. Do you do follow-up work if the surgery does not meet our agreed-upon expectations?

7. If a follow-up procedure is required, will I be charged?

8. Who assists you with surgery, and what are their qualifications?

9. What will be the total cost of my facelift procedure?

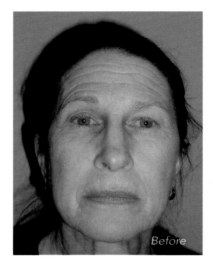
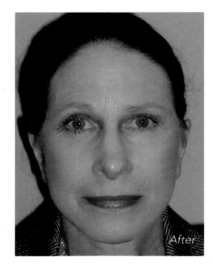
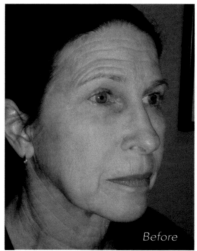
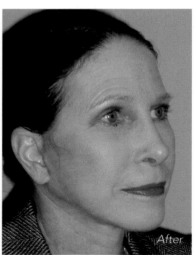

Facelift with modified deep chemical peel

emergency were to arise. Organizations that accredit surgical centers include those listed below.

- Accreditation Association for Ambulatory Health Care (AAAHC)
- American Association for Accreditation of Ambulatory Surgery Facilities (AAAASF)
- Joint Commission for Accreditation of Healthcare Organizations (JCAHO)

Studies have shown that accredited facilities staffed with professional anesthesia personnel are not only safe but can actually minimize complications such as infection. Specialized facilities offer comfort, privacy, and safety.

Beyond asking about accreditation, also visit the suite itself and observe its staff. Does the staff treat you with respect? Are they helpful, and do they respond to your questions with courtesy? Do you get the sense that you will be in good hands if your surgery is performed there?

If the meeting goes well with the doctor and all your questions are answered, and if you are satisfied with both the doctor and the surgical suite, then you are ready to schedule your facelift.

CHAPTER THREE

Preparing for Facelift Surgery

3

Preparing for Facelift Surgery

Amazing advances have been made in the field of cosmetic surgery, and cosmetic surgeries are now available to many of us. This, along with extensive media coverage about cosmetic surgery, tends to make us think of this surgery as being only a minor inconvenience we undergo to get the results we want. However, it is important to remember that this is still surgery, and it needs to be taken seriously. The more you know about the surgery and what to expect, the better prepared you'll be.

As the date for your surgery nears, you will need to make some preparations. You will be given instructions by your surgeon.

Standard Lab Tests

Your surgeon wants to make sure you are in good overall health before proceeding with cosmetic surgery. Accordingly, he or she will likely ask you to undergo some routine lab tests. These are usually done a few weeks prior to your surgery and may be coordinated with your primary care provider.

Complete Blood Count

Through a *complete blood count (CBC)*, your doctor will check your white blood cells, platelets, and hemoglobin, all of which play important roles during surgery. White blood cells help you fight off infection. A normal platelet level reduces your chances of excessive bleeding and bruising. Hemoglobin carries oxygen to your body's organs and tissues; a normal hemoglobin level will aid you in healing.

Electrocardiogram

An *electrocardiogram (ECG* or *EKG)*, which measures electrical activity of the heart, is used to check for heart disease, irregular heartbeats, and evidence of past heart attacks. Your doctor will probably order this test for you if you are over age forty or if you have a history of heart disease. Your surgeon wants to be sure that you have no heart conditions that would make cosmetic surgery inadvisable.

Chest X-ray

Most cosmetic surgeons do not routinely order chest X-rays prior to performing facelifts. However, if you are a smoker, a chest X-ray may be ordered to rule out lung disease and any problems with the respiratory tract, heart, and lymph glands.

Medications You'll Need

Pain Medication

Most individuals who have facelifts report having little postsurgical pain, but your surgeon will likely give you a prescription for pain medication, to be filled prior to your surgery. Or your doctor may give you pain medication tablets to take home after your surgery is completed.

Antibiotics

You will likely be given a prescription for an antibiotic, which is to be taken for several days after surgery to prevent infection.

Antiviral Medication

You will probably be asked to start taking antiviral medication the night before your procedure.

Other Prescriptions

Your doctor may also prescribe other medications, depending on the procedure and your needs. These include such drugs as antihistamines, decongestants, anti-inflammatory drugs, stool softeners, vitamins, ointments, and sedatives.

> "*What type of facelift should you have? Discuss your wishes as your cosmetic surgeon examines your face. The two of you can then decide which procedures will give you the best outcome.*"
>
> —David Ellis, M.D.

Medications to Avoid before Surgery

You'll be asked to avoid certain medications, including aspirin and aspirin products, prior to your surgery. Aspirin thins the blood and can increase the risk of bleeding during or after the surgery. Your surgeon will give your detailed instructions about this, including this list of products to avoid:

Advil	Dristan Decongestant
Aleve	Empirin
Anacin	Excedrin
Alka-Seltzer	Ibuprofen
Aspirin	Liquiprin
Arthritis Pain Formula	Medipren
Aspergum	Midol 200
Bayer	Motrin
Bufferin	Nuprin
Dolobid	Pepto-Bismol

This list is not intended to be comprehensive. Your surgeon will advise you on which medications to avoid.

Supplements to Avoid

Just as aspirin can promote bleeding, so can some supplements or herbal preparations. You will likely be asked to avoid such supplements as vitamin E and various herbal medications, such as St. John's Wort and ginseng.

Avoid Alcohol

Your surgeon will instruct you to avoid alcohol for two weeks prior to your surgery, and for at least two weeks. Alcohol thins the blood and can promote bleeding.

Arrange for a Caregiver

Prior to your surgery, you will need to arrange for an adult caregiver. This individual will drive you to and from the surgical center. Your mental sharpness will be affected by the anesthesia, and you will not be permitted to drive immediately after a facelift.

The caregiver should be prepared to spend the first twenty-four hours with you after your procedure. The caregiver can help you with such things as going to the bathroom, taking medications, and preparing meals. If you don't have a relative or friend who is available, your surgeon or his staff often will have the names of nurses or nurse's aides who are available for such duties.

Some surgeons have a staffed recovery facility for their patients or work with a hotel and private duty nurses to provide care.

The Pre-op Office Visit

Your surgeon may ask you to come to the office prior to the date of your procedure to discuss post operative care and necessary supplies, as well as future office visits. At this time, he or she will make sure all paperwork has been completed and answer any additional questions you may have about the upcoming procedure. Pre-op photos also may be taken during this visit.

The Night before Your Surgery

Fasting

If the procedure you're having will require anesthesia, it's important that you not eat or drink anything after midnight the night before your surgery. Why is this important? It takes six to eight hours for your stomach to empty itself of food after you've eaten. If you have food in your stomach when you undergo anesthesia, there is a risk of aspirating, vomiting of food particles into the trachea (airway) or lungs during surgery. This can lead to infections, chronic cough, obstruction in the lungs, or a serious condition called *aspiration pneumonia.* The anesthesia provider will cancel the procedure if fasting is violated.

Wash with Antibacterial Soap

Your doctor may tell you to cleanse your face with a prescription surgical soap or antibacterial soap the night before your surgery and the morning of your procedure. This cleansing will help reduce the chance of infection from the bacteria on your skin.

Day 2 of Your Surgery

Depending on the instructions your surgeon and anesthesia provider gave you, you may be able to take routine prescription drugs on the morning of your surgery. In some cases, you may be advised to take them with only a sip of water.

Wash your hair if you didn't the night before, and apply the prescription soap if so directed by your doctor. Do not apply skin moisturizers, conditioners, makeup, perfume, or hair spray on the morning of your surgery. Ask your doctor if it's okay to use deodorant.

Wear a shirt that you can unbutton or unzip to take off, rather than one that needs to be lifted over your head. It's also best to wear slip-on shoes so that you do not need to bend over to tie them after your procedure; bending over increases the blood flow to your face and could damage the delicate tissues that are healing.

You will be asked to remove all jewelry, rings, and watches, as well as contact lenses. It is recommended that you leave these and other valuables at home.

Arriving at the Surgery Center

When you arrive at the surgery center, you'll complete any required administrative paperwork, including an informed consent form, which you'll be asked to sign if you haven't already done so. (See chapter 2.)

Once your paperwork is completed, you will be asked to change into a hospital gown. Your hair will need to be pulled away from your face; it can be secured with elastic bands or clips.

At this point, a nurse may give you a sedative to help you relax and will insert an IV line in your arm or perhaps in the top of your hand. The medical team will use the IV to administer anesthesia along with any other drugs given during your facelift procedure. If you have any personal items with you, you can give them to the caregiver who accompanies you or ask to have them put in a secure place at the surgery center.

Meeting with Your Surgeon

Prior to your surgical procedure, you'll meet with your surgeon. This will be an opportunity to ask any last-minute questions. At this time, the surgeon may place surgical markings on your face; these markings will guide him or her in making incisions. For example, the surgeon might mark the creases on your forehead and around your mouth and mark the bands of tissue on your neck. The surgeon may also circle pockets of fat to be removed or repositioned or mark your eyelid crease.

Meeting with the Anesthesiologist

You may also receive a brief visit from the anesthesiologist during the preparations for surgery. He or she will verify that you haven't had anything to eat or drink other than a few sips of water with any necessary medication. Your anesthesiologist will also check that you haven't been taking any of the medications your surgeon instructed you to avoid. A quick review of your medical history may also be part of this visit. The anesthesiologist may ask you about certain medical conditions, any allergies to food or medications, and whether you or a family member have ever had any allergic reactions to anesthesia. What do food allergies have to do with anesthesia? Some anesthetics contain components of foods, such as eggs, so it's important to inform the anesthesiologist of any food allergies. And although adverse reactions to anesthesia are rare, they can run in families. Even though you've already included this information in your medical history, it's important to review it with the anesthesiologist. This review is done to ensure your safety during your procedure, so be sure to bring up anything you may have forgotten to include in your history. If you have any last-minute questions about anesthesia or pain control during the procedure, ask the anesthesiologist.

What Type of Anesthesia Will Be Used?

During your pre-op visit, you likely will have discussed with your surgeon the different types of anesthesia. The type of anesthesia used to keep you pain-free during the procedure should be directly related to the type of procedure to be performed and be administered by either an anesthesiologist (M.D.) or a Certified Registered Nurse Anesthetist (CRNA).

If you feel somewhat nervous about being "put under" with anesthesia, you're not alone. It's common to experience some anxiety about undergoing anesthesia. However, you should know that anesthesia is safer than ever before. In fact, a 1999 report from the Institute of Medicine states that anesthesia is fifty times safer than it was in the early 1980s. What makes it so much safer today? It's due to improvements in the drugs used in anesthesia, in the education of anesthesia providers, in technology, and in the techniques

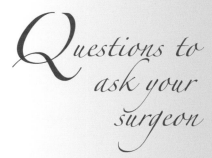

Questions to ask your surgeon

1. Which lab tests will I need?

2. Is it okay to take routine medications the day of my surgery?

3. What kind of anesthesia will be used during my surgery?

4. What are the side effects of the surgery?

5. Do I need to use a special soap or shampoo the morning of my surgery?

6. Should I combine facial procedures or have them done separately?

used for monitoring patients during surgery. The anesthesiologist or surgeon makes the final decision about the type and level of anesthesia you receive.

Local Anesthesia

Local anesthesia involves an injection to numb a small portion of your body, preventing you from feeling any pain in that area. Local anesthesia, when used alone, leaves you fully alert and allows you to breathe on your own. Local anesthetics wouldn't be used alone for standard facelifts; however, some surgeons performing mini facelifts use local anesthesia along with an oral sedative. The agents in local anesthetics remain in the body for a very short time and do not cause feelings of grogginess. There are limits to the amount of local anesthesia that can be used, but this type of anesthesia can be useful for more limited procedures of shorter duration. Your surgeon, rather than an anesthesia provider, may administer this anesthesia.

Sedation Anesthesia

Sedation anesthesia puts you into a light sleep with a combination of sedatives and pain relievers. Local anesthetic is often used to provide additional pain relief. With sedation anesthesia, you can breathe on your own, so there is no need for a breathing tube. Sedation anesthesia does not remain in the body long, and you can expect to feel normal within a few hours after surgery. Sedation anesthesia may also be referred to as monitored anesthesia care (MAC) or twilight sedation.

Sedation anesthesia may be administered in varying levels: minimal, moderate, and deep.

Minimal sedation: With this level of sedation, you remain awake but relaxed during your procedure, and you don't feel pain or discomfort. Your memory of the procedure isn't affected with minimal sedation.

Moderate sedation: You'll feel drowsy and may sleep through portions of or all of your procedure with moderate sedation. However, you can be easily awakened if touched or spoken to. You may or may not remember what happens during your procedure.

Deep sedation: You'll sleep through your procedure and most likely won't remember much about it.

General Anesthesia

Any anesthesia that uses a breathing tube is automatically classified as a *general anesthesia*. Similar to sedation, there are different levels of general anesthesia, depending on the procedure. Facial plastic surgery procedures do not require the deep levels of anesthesia necessary for removing a gall bladder or replacing a hip. Lighter medication and breathing tubes have been shown to be both safe and effective. Newer medications, such as propofol, provide the safety of controlled breathing through breathing tube intubation with the short-acting, pleasant recovery provided by the intravenous medication.

How You'll Be Monitored during Your Surgery

During your surgery, the medical team will monitor your vital signs. A cuff on your arm will monitor your blood pressure. A pulse oximeter, clipped to the tip of your forefinger, will measure the level of oxygen in your blood. For your safety and comfort during combined procedures, the surgical team will likely provide you with compression boots (to avoid blood clots), body cushioning, and warming blankets.

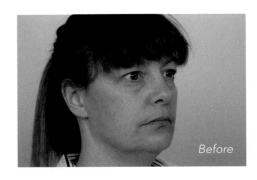
Before

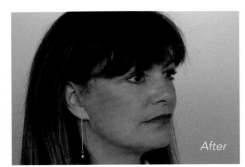
After

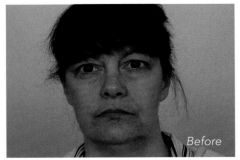
Before

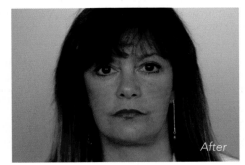
After

Facelift, eyelid lift

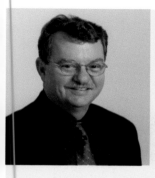

William Truswell, M.D.
Facial Plastic Surgeon
Northampton, MA

What do you find most rewarding about your work? There's a great deal that's enjoyable about it. From a personal perspective, I enjoy the artistry of facial cosmetic surgery, and the fact that my work is a creative endeavor in medicine is something that I find extremely rewarding. Facial cosmetic surgery is a "happy" specialty. The patients are in good health and are motivated. We know from the outcomes that we are making improvements in people's lives.

Describe the types of patients you see. What procedures are they seeking? Interestingly, for the last five to ten years we've seen patients coming in at younger and younger ages for rejuvenation surgery. And we have found that with the younger patient we can produce results that are much more natural and easier to maintain. I also see a trend in patients seeking minimally invasive procedures—everything from Botox to thread lifts. There's been a big push for procedures that decrease the amount of downtime, are relatively affordable, and have good results.

What has been one of the biggest changes in cosmetic surgery in recent years? I would have to say the more minimally invasive procedures. Also, laser technology over the last ten years has been amazing. We can use lasers for such procedures as skin resurfacing as well as for removing excess hair and tiny blood vessels, such as those in the nose.

What procedures are you doing now that you didn't do five years ago? Well, certainly the thread lifts. In 2004, the FDA approved the barb threads. Previously, we were doing thread lifts by doing a suspension of the fat pads on the cheeks. The threads do a better job of lifting and produce longer-lasting results. With the threads, you're spreading the suspension over the length of the thread as opposed to suspending the tissue in one location. It gives a better result.

How have patients responded to these procedures? The response from patients is good. In fact, it's patients who are driving the demand for these services. Of course, the press plays a role. People learn about new procedures from television shows and women's magazines. Then they come into our office, asking for these procedures—such as Thermage and Restylane, the wrinkle filler.

What new developments are yet to come in facial cosmetic surgery? I think what you're going to see in the future is permanent injectable fillers used to fill creases and wrinkles. This type of filler will give more volume to the face without the need for implants. There will also probably be more developments with lasers, which will produce better collagen reproduction and quicker healing from resurfacing.

Describe one of the most memorable patients you've had recently. It would be a young girl who was in an automobile accident and hit her nose on the steering wheel and fractured all the bones of her midface. Both her nose and her cheeks were flattened. I reconstructed her midface—brought her nose up and inserted cheek implants. I also did some scar revision. A few weeks later she came into my office, dressed up and wearing makeup. She looked very pretty. That was a great feeling.

CHAPTER FOUR

The Standard Facelift

4

The Standard Facelift

Most of us have similar beliefs about what constitutes beauty. In the United States, the ideal attractive facial features are generally considered to be symmetry, high cheekbones, and an angular jawline. However, even those with ideal features experience a change in their facial structure as they age. The same holds true for all of us. But today, more Americans are choosing to defy the effects of aging through cosmetic surgery, namely, the facelift. No longer is such cosmetic surgery only for the rich and famous. For many, it is an extension of wellness and feeling good about oneself.

With the extensive marketing you are exposed to today, you have likely heard about different types of facial rejuvenation, and the one you're probably heard the most about is the standard facelift. It has become a commonly performed cosmetic procedure in the United States.

What Is a Standard Facelift?

The SMAS Facelift

A standard facelift, known as a *rhytidectomy* in medical terms, is a procedure in which the loose skin on the cheeks and neck, along with the underlying sagging muscles, are lifted and tightened. The most common standard lift is a *SMAS facelift*. SMAS refers to *subcutaneous musculoaponeurotic system*, the soft tissues that lie under our facial skin; these tissues consist of fat, a layer of connective tissue, and muscles. As we age, these underlying structures begin to sag, pulling our skin along with them. The fat pads in our cheeks slide downward, our cheeks become hollow, and we develop jowls and creases.

The SMAS facelift is longer lasting and produces a more natural look than a lift in which only loose skin is pulled tight. Skin-only facelifts, first introduced decades ago, are rarely used today. The SMAS facelift is sometimes referred to as a two-layer facelift, because surgeons do just that: they lift two layers. The first layer is skin and the second is the SMAS.

Are You a Candidate for a Facelift?

The best way to determine if you're a good candidate for a facelift is to talk with a cosmetic surgeon. When you understand what facelifts can and can't do, and after you have undergone an examination by the surgeon, you and the surgeon can decide whether a facelift is right for you, and, if so, what type of facelift. Following are basic characteristics that make some people more suitable than others for a facelift.

Are Your Expectations Realistic?

Cosmetic surgery produces improvements—not perfection. It's important that you have realistic expectations about the improvements cosmetic surgery can and cannot make.

Will You Be a Compliant Patient?

The patients who have the best outcomes with their cosmetic surgery are those who carry out their responsibilities. These include following presurgery instructions (such as not smoking and avoiding certain medications) and postoperative instructions (such as resting and taking it easy while they are healing).

Is Your Body Weight Stable?

A significant weight loss or weight gain will affect the results of a facelift. If you lose more than ten to fifteen pounds after surgery, your skin will sag again. If you plan to lose weight, lose it before you get a facelift. People who are overweight can have successful facelifts, although their improvements aren't as successful as they would be if the patients were in a normal weight range. The deeper the facelift, the less weight is a factor.

Is Your Overall Health Good?

For any type of surgery, you should be in good overall health. Your body needs to be healthy to both tolerate the stress of surgery and to heal properly afterward. If you have a chronic disease, such as uncontrolled diabetes or heart disease, you should be cautioned about surgery because you have a greater anesthetic risk. Surgeons often arrange for these individuals to have an anesthesia consultation prior to scheduling surgery.

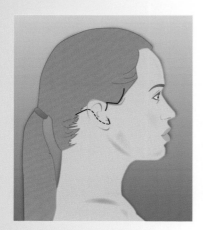

Standard facelift incision for women

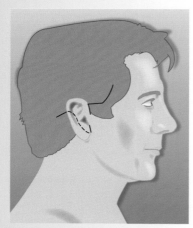

Standard facelift incision for men

If you have an autoimmune disease that affects your face, such as lupus or scleroderma, you should not have a facelift. Likewise, if you're taking medication to suppress your immune system, you might not be a good candidate for the surgery, because the medication can slow the healing process. Before planning any surgery, talk with your surgeon about any health issues or worries that you have.

Are You a Nonsmoker?

Smoking and cosmetic surgery are a bad combination. Smoking can impair healing, and smokers risk loss of skin, or skin death, because smoking causes a restriction in the flow of blood through their blood vessels. These delicate vessels may be stretched and pulled during the facelift, and, whereas normal blood vessels stretch and then recover, smokers' vessels could shut off entirely. Smokers can have successful facelifts, but it's imperative that they stop smoking several weeks before and after the procedure. Still, the best candidate for a facelift is someone who doesn't smoke at all.

Undergoing a SMAS Facelift

It typically takes between two to four hours for a surgeon to perform a SMAS facelift. The surgeon follows these basic steps:

- The surgeon makes an incision, separating the skin from the underlying tissue. The placement of incisions varies, though incisions are commonly in the hairline from the temple to the top of the ear, vertically in front of and behind the ear, and horizontally in the hairline and under the chin.
- Excess fat may be suctioned away.
- The SMAS is elevated and repositioned so its back edge overlaps the surrounding tissue, or it is folded over itself. The shaping of these underlying muscles creates a more youthful appearance.
- The skin is redraped and excess is trimmed.
- The skin is reattached using a combination of skin clips, staples, removable sutures, and dissolvable sutures. The surgeon decides which of these are most appropriate and closes the incision accordingly.

When surgeons perform a neck lift, they not only lift the SMAS layer, but they also tighten the platysma muscle, which extends from the lower jaw to the collarbone. Neck

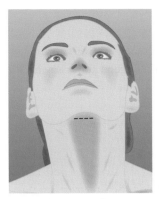
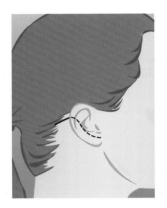
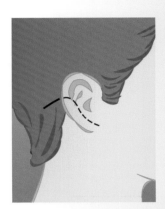

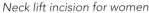

Neck lift incision for women   Neck lift incision for men

lifts are part of both standard facelifts and deep-plane facelifts. By making incisions behind the ears and one tiny incision under the chin, surgeons are able to lift the neck tissues and remove excess skin, essentially "resculpting" the neck. The neck lift is also referred to as a *platysma lift* or a *platysmaplasty.*

Faster Healing with Platelet Gel

Just prior to closing your incisions, your surgeon may place *platelet gel* under your facial skin. Platelet gel, a newer tool used by surgeons, is harvested from your own blood. This gel stimulates the body's own healing abilities, and because the gel is so concentrated, it also acts as wound sealant or tissue glue.

How is platelet gel acquired? Prior to surgery, approximately 45 cubic centimeters, or 1.5 ounces, of blood is drawn from your arm. The blood is spun in a centrifuge, which separates its different components. The rich platelet gel is then combined with another compound and the mixture is sprayed under the skin before incisions are closed.

In addition to stimulating the healing process, the gel eliminates the need for some dressings and drains. It also reduces the incidence of complications such as a *hematoma* (a pool of blood under the skin) or a *seroma* (a pool of fluid under the skin), and reduces bruising and swelling.

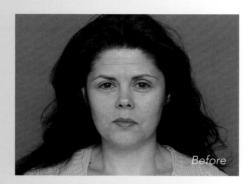

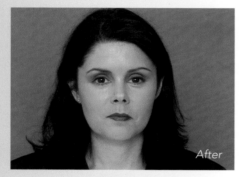

Standard facelift, brow lift, eyelid lift, and laser skin resurfacing

Drainage Tubes

In some cases, the surgeon will insert thin drainage tubes in the incisions behind your ears to drain away excess fluids that may collect under the skin. A small suction bulb is attached to the end of the tubes and fluid is suctioned into the bulbs. These tubes are needed because when the face is lifted and repositioned, vessels between the skin and deeper tissues are disrupted, and serum—the clear liquid part of blood—can accumulate. If this accumulation is more than your body can reabsorb, you may develop a seroma, which can impede healing. Drainage tubes prevent this from occurring.

If you have drains inserted, the collection bulbs will be concealed within your clothing and you will be told how to care for them at home. Your drains will be removed on your first visit to your doctor after your surgery, usually a day later.

After the surgeon closes the incisions, your head is wrapped with gauze and a stretch bandage that goes under your chin and over the top of your head. Your face is left exposed. This bandage stabilizes the face and holds the flaps in place overnight. This bandage is usually removed the next day.

After Your Facelift

Once your facelift has been completed, you will be moved to a recovery room where you will continue to be monitored. You will be checked to ensure you are recovering from the anesthesia and are experiencing no complications. Nausea and other untoward effects such as feeling cold are easily avoided today, but you will feel a little groggy from the anesthetic. However, because of the advent of short-acting intravenous anesthesic agents, such as propofol, whether you received sedation or general anesthesia, you will be up and walking in a short time. Some people may complain of a mild sore throat if a breathing tube was used.

You will probably feel well enough to go home after an hour or two in the recovery room. At this point you can be driven home by your caregiver or taken to your recovery environment.

Your surgeon will schedule a follow-up appointment with you.

If your surgeon inserted any drainage tubes, these will usually be removed during this follow-up visit. The surgeon will also remove bandages and examine your incisions.

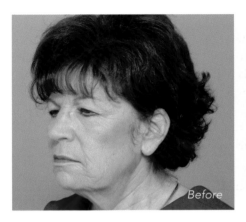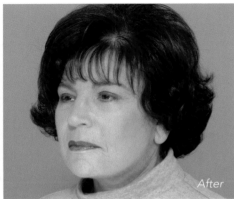

Standard facelift, brow lift, eyelid lift, soft tissue filler in nasolabial folds

Typically, the surgeon will remove metal clips or external sutures several days after surgery.

Side Effects

Side effects of facelift surgery are normal, temporary, and to be expected. Be patient in the first few weeks. Your final result won't be apparent for weeks or months, once all side effects have subsided.

Swelling and Bruising

After a standard facelift, your face will be swollen and bruised. Swelling should peak in two to three days, and then begin to subside. It will take several months for all swelling to dissipate; however, this swelling is usually very subtle and not noticeable to others. Some bruising might linger up to two to three weeks, but by the third week, you should be looking and feeling much better. You should feel comfortable going back to work in two weeks.

Numbness

You may have some temporary numbness, which typically occurs around the ears and in the cheeks. It might take several weeks, or even a few months, for you to regain total sensation. Only in very rare cases does any numbness remain for a longer period of time.

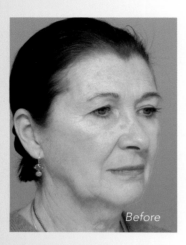
Before

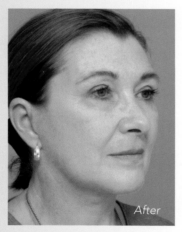
After

Standard facelift, brow lift, eyelid lift

Stiffness and Discomfort

As mentioned earlier, most patients do not have pain after a facelift; however, you will probably experience some discomfort and a tightness or stiffness in your face. These symptoms are mild and will gradually disappear within a week or two.

Low Mood

Don't be surprised if you have a mild case of the "blues" in the days immediately following your surgery. This is common. Being aware of this will help you cope with any temporary mood swings. For the experienced surgeon, facial plastic surgery issues such as patient low mood are minimized by providing a support network of patient coordinators, nurses, patient referrals, and frequent office visits with the surgeon.

Incision Line Visibility

Incisions made in front of the ear generally heal with minimal scarring. If you're a woman, you may have chosen to let your hair grow longer on the sides; the hair can help to hide the healing incisions in front of the ears until the scar matures. Incisions made behind the ear can sometimes leave scars, because the skin behind the ear is thicker. But this area is usually covered with hair and is not noticeable. Most scars will fade within three to twelve months.

Remember, even perfect incision lines can be temporarily visible. Certain skin types will have reddening on any healing incision line, which can make them temporarily apparent. Incision lines can be easily camouflaged within a few weeks.

The hairline will be altered by incision placement. Incisions hidden inside hairlines will move the hairline up. Incisions on the edge of hairlines will preserve the entire hairline.

Potential Complications

As explained earlier, side effects are normal and to be expected, and their symptoms diminish on their own. However, complications are *not* normal, and usually require treatment. The overall incidence of complications with facial cosmetic surgery is rare, about 1 or 2 percent, according to the American Society of Plastic Surgeons. Still, it is important to be aware of potential complications.

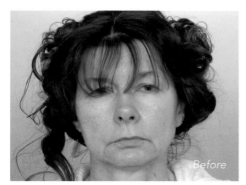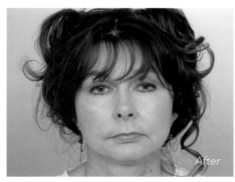

Standard facelift, neck lift, upper and lower eyelid lift, brow lift, laser skin resurfacing around the mouth

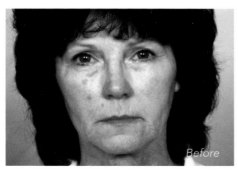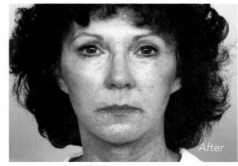

Standard facelift, neck lift, lower and upper eyelid lift, laser skin resurfacing around the eyes and mouth

Infection

With modern surgical techniques and antibiotics, postsurgical infection is rare; however, it is still possible. Infection typically occurs when bacteria enters the body through incision sites, sutures, or drains. For this reason, antibiotics are usually given during and following a surgical procedure.

Hematoma

A hematoma, a pool of blood that collects within the tissue under flaps of skin, usually occurs within the first twenty-four hours after surgery. If, after your surgery, you have swelling and significant pain in one spot, call your surgeon immediately. It could be an indication of a hematoma. Surgeons treat these by draining the blood that has accumulated. When hematomas are treated early, they usually do not cause serious tissue damage. However, if a hematoma is left untreated, it can result in the death of the skin tissue.

Necrosis

Also known as skin death, *necrosis* is usually caused by insufficient oxygen reaching tissues. This complication is rare, but can occur after surgery in which flaps of skin are separated from their blood supply. The risk of necrosis increases with significant swelling. Smokers are more likely to experience this complication.

Seroma

A seroma is a collection of fluid, serum, that collects under the skin. It's the same type of fluid you would see in a blister. A seroma can become infected if it does not dissipate. A seroma may dissipate on its own, or the surgeon may need to drain it. Since most seromas occur within the first few days after surgery, it's often a condition that the surgeon would discover during a follow-up examination.

Nerve Injury

A surgical procedure can manipulate certain nerves, both sensory (touch/feel) and motor (movement). All facial procedures produce temporary numbness, as discussed as a side effect. The areas affected are not used as sensory organs, such as your fingers, so the numbness tends not to bother most people. Rarely, sensation does not return and this numbness becomes a complication. Injury to motor nerves is very rare, 0.5 percent, and is usually temporary, with a return of full movement and sensation within a few months. Signs that numbness will recover are tingling, itching, and quick sensation.

Spitting Suture

A spitting suture is not a serious complication, and can occur weeks or months after any type of surgery. It happens when the body treats an absorbable suture as a foreign object and tries to reject it rather than absorb it. This will result in the suture being pushed to the skin's surface. The suture may appear to be a pimple or a blackhead. If this should occur, your surgeon can easily remove the suture; no incision is required.

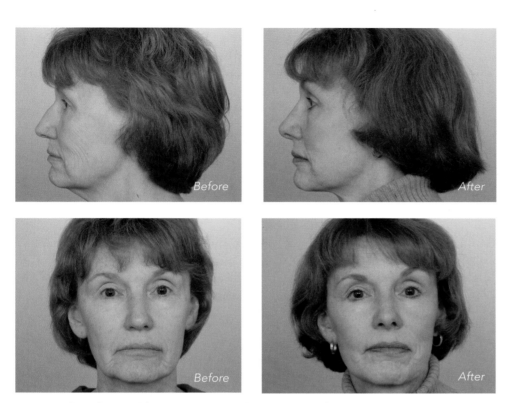

Standard facelift, neck lift, nose reshaping, laser skin resurfacing around the mouth

Slow Healing

Another possible complication is slow healing. This occurs most often in smokers, due to restricted flow of blood to vessels, or in patients with other medical issues.

Ear Distortion

Excessive skin tightening when suturing to the ear incision site can cause this problem. Experienced surgeons spend a great deal of time detailing ear incisions to avoid this complication.

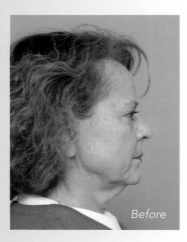

Before

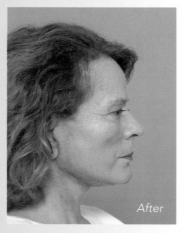

After

Standard facelift with midface lifted with threads

Hair Loss and Hairline Changes

Hair loss is related to skin-only facelifts where the skin is pulled too tightly. This can also be a complication with smokers. Hairlines are often affected in facial plastic surgery; consequently, experienced surgeons are able to plan and predict any hairline alterations. Poor planning can lead to an unauthentic hairline.

When to Contact Your Surgeon

If any complications should arise, you should contact your surgeon's office even if you're not sure what the complications mean. Conditions that require you to contact him or her immediately include:

- Signs of infection. If you have a temperature of a degree and a half over your normal temperature, or if you notice pus or inflammation at the incision site or have significant pain, call your doctor immediately. Usually signs of infection do not occur within the first five days after the procedure.
- Excessive bleeding. You will have a little bleeding after your surgery, but it should be minimal and short-lived. If this isn't the case, let your doctor know right away.
- Hematoma. If you have increasing pain in one part of your face, it could be a hematoma. In most cases, you would not actually see a hematoma, because your head would probably still be wrapped in bandages.
- Seroma. This is a painless condition. If you were to have a seroma, you wouldn't see fluid under the skin, but you would likely feel swelling behind the ear.

Recovery

Because of the nature of facial cosmetic surgery, it is common for a patient to have a professional caregiver for the first night. Providing someone, such as a nurse, who has experience in knowing what "things should look like" creates peace of mind for you and your family. Rarely is medical monitoring necessary but peace of mind has tremendous value. Retreats or recovery hotels are common and provide a sophisticated total environment over an extended period of time, if desired. They also offer privacy, pampering, and convenience.

If you will be going home soon after your procedure, you may want to ask your doctor for the name of a professional caregiver who can stay with you for at least the first night.

Your surgeon will recommend that once you're home or in your suite you spend the first few hours resting, keeping your head elevated on your bed, couch, or recliner. Here are some tips for your initial recovery:

- Get plenty of rest. Sit in a chair during your waking hours.
- Avoid bending over in the days immediately following your facelift. When you bend over, blood rushes to your face and can potentially damage the delicate tissues that are healing.
- Avoid heavy lifting.
- Move slowly and avoid turning your head sharply; such sudden movements can damage the sutures.
- Sleep only on your back for the first several nights after your surgery to avoid additional swelling. This instruction varies among surgeons.
- When lying down, keep your head elevated for at least the first three days to avoid swelling in the face.
- Keep medications and a glass of water nearby.
- Avoid aspirin and other blood-thinning drugs.
- Clear any medications with your doctor.
- Avoid alcohol for two weeks, especially if you're taking pain or sleep medications, unless otherwise instructed by your surgeon.
- Refrain from smoking.
- Follow the diet guidelines your surgeon has recommended. Recommendations often include bland foods the first day after surgery to avoid any stomach upset. Afterward, you can likely resume normal eating habits. Eat nutritious meals and drink plenty of water.
- Apply cold cloths, dipped in ice water and wrung out, as directed to help reduce swelling.
- Your surgeon may give you instructions to apply a silicone gel to your incisions after sutures are removed. This gel can help scars fade more quickly, and it can help minimize scarring as well.

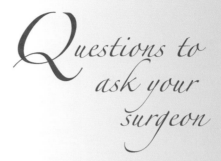

Questions to ask your surgeon

1. Which procedure is best for me?
2. What kind of preoperative evaluation do I need?
3. In which surgical facility will my facelift be performed?
4. What kind of anesthesia is used?
5. Is there much postsurgical pain?
6. Where will the incisions be?
7. How long is the recovery period?
8. How soon can I wear glasses?
9. When can I go back to work?
10. When can I wear my contacts?

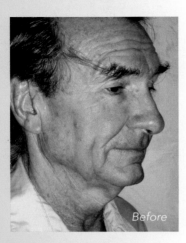

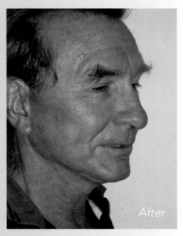

Facelift with modified deep chemical peel

Bathing and Grooming

Usually, you can shower or bathe within a day or two of surgery. Ask your doctor when you can do so, and when you can resume other activities, such as brushing your teeth. Men are typically asked to refrain from shaving near their incision lines until instructed.

Returning to Work

Usually, you can return to work after seven to ten days, as long as your work does not require heavy lifting or other strenuous activity. Some people return earlier, some take a little longer.

Going Out in Public

Most people feel "presentable" in public within two weeks. Ask you doctor when you can begin applying makeup again. Usually, you can do so within five to ten days.

Exercising

You shouldn't exercise for about two weeks after a facelift, because it could cause swelling and bleeding. After you get approval from your doctor and begin exercising again, ease into it for the first few weeks, and closely monitor any signs of swelling. Stop rigorous exercise if you notice swelling and call your doctor.

Resuming Sexual Relations

Most doctors recommend that you abstain from sexual relations for the same period of time that you refrain from exercising.

Protecting Yourself from Sun Exposure

You want to be especially careful in your first year after surgery, because any scars that are exposed to sunlight could become permanently darkened. When you are outdoors, make sure you protect your skin by applying sunscreen with an SPF rating of at least 15, and preferably one that is higher. The sunscreen should be applied thirty minutes before you go out. If you have received a laser treatment, wear a hat, as well.

How Long Will a Facelift Last?

This question does not have just one answer that fits everyone. The length of time a facelift will last varies, but it generally lasts from four to twelve years. The longevity is affected by several factors. The older you are, the fewer years your lift will last. Another factor is the degree of tissue laxity and skin thickness. A patient with little elasticity left in the skin will need a tightening procedure sooner than a person with greater elasticity. The results won't last as long for a person with what is referred to as a "heavy face"; this usually includes men, who have heavier, coarser skin.

Other longevity factors include your overall health, the type of lift you've had, and your personal opinion about the outcome of the lift. One person may feel happy about the results of a facelift for many years; another may return to the surgeon after only a few years, asking about a "mini tuck," a minor procedure to refresh a facelift.

If you have skin damage from sun exposure or other factors, resurfacing procedures can help a facelift last longer. They are described in depth in a later chapter.

If you lose a lot of weight after your facelift, you will be at a higher risk for recurrent sagging. However, if you maintain a healthful weight, don't smoke, and take good care of yourself and your skin, your facelift can last from seven to twelve years.

Revision Facelifts

In most cases, a revision facelift is performed on an individual who had a facelift a decade ago, enjoyed the results, and would like a renewal or further rejuvenation. SMAS techniques can usually be repeated once for subtle improvement without producing excessive tightening.

Combining Facelifts with Other Procedures

Because all of the face ages at the same rate, to effectively rejuvenate the face, often it should be approached as a unit. A facelift accomplishes the lower face rejuvenation; however, a brow lift or eyelid lift may also be necessary to balance the face. When procedures are not combined, a beautiful facelift could create bunching, pleats at the sides of the eyes or, at a minimum, an unbalanced appearance. Because combining procedures does not add significantly to the recovery time, it is best to have these procedures performed at the same time.

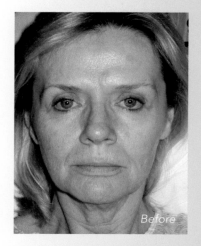
Before

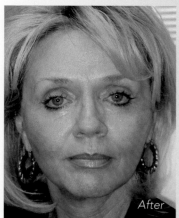
After

Standard facelift

CHAPTER FIVE

The Deep-Plane Lift

5

The Deep-Plane Lift

*J*ust as advancements have been made in other areas of medicine, advancements have been made in the field of cosmetic surgery, and the future promises the development of even more procedures to rejuvenate the face. One of the newer techniques in face-lifting is the *deep-plane lift*, which was developed in the early 1990s. This procedure is more complex than a standard SMAS facelift, and facial plastic surgeons who perform the procedure usually require special training. Presently, only a small number of surgeons—perhaps only several dozen—are specifically trained in the procedure.

What Is a Deep-Plane Facelift?

A modification of the standard facelift, the deep-plane facelift involves elevating and repositioning the drooping facial structures—muscles and fat—that lie in the layer (plane) below the SMAS layer. This facelift is effective in restoring the midface—the fat pads in the cheeks are lifted, resulting in more natural contours of the cheeks and softening of the nasolabial folds.

The deep-plane technique can be modified to include only the midface, from under the eyes to the jawbone, or adapted to an even smaller area for a mini-lift. If you are younger and do not see signs of aging in your neck, you and your plastic surgeon might consider one of these options.

Are You a Candidate for a Deep-Plane Facelift?

In general, any candidate for a standard facelift is also a candidate for a deep-plane facelift. Some surgeons believe that a deep-plane facelift may be a better choice for smokers than a standard facelift, since the deep-plane area has a more ample blood supply and is more resistant to smoking complications.

Are Your Expectations Realistic?

If your goal is to look younger and fresher—more as you did ten or twenty years ago—then you will probably be pleased with the results of a deep-plane facelift.

Will You Be a Compliant Patient?

Compliant doesn't mean "uninformed." It's important to ask questions when there's something you don't understand. You should choose an experienced surgeon who welcomes your questions and whom you trust.

He or she will give you detailed instructions for before and after surgery. Question anything that seems unclear, so that when the time comes you can follow these instructions to the letter.

Is Your Body Weight Stable?

Body weight is less an issue with a deep-plane facelift than with a standard facelift, which is done at or above the fat layer. If you lose a lot of weight after a standard facelift, your facial tissues will sag again.

Since a deep-plane lift tightens tissues below the fat layer, losing weight (ten to twenty-five pounds) will not affect the results. The skin will remain smoothly draped, since it is not bearing the weight of the underlying tissues.

You don't need to worry about stabilizing your weight before a deep-plane facelift unless you are planning a drastic weight loss, over 100 pounds. If this is the case, discuss the timing of your facelift with your plastic surgeon.

Is Your Overall Health Good?

Remember that you will be undergoing a three- to five-hour procedure. You won't be aware of what's happening, but your body will. You should be healthy enough to tolerate the surgery and heal quickly afterward. It is normal to have pre-procedure medical screening by your internist to define your health status objectively.

Discuss with your surgeon any chronic conditions, such as diabetes or heart disease, that might put you at risk under anesthesia. Do you have any conditions that may interfere

> "Younger people have more options today for reversing the signs of aging through facial cosmetic surgery. You don't have to wait until you look old to make changes."
> —Neil A. Gordon, M.D.

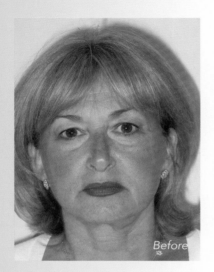

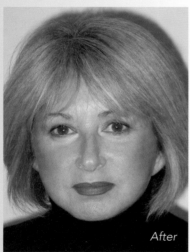

Deep-plane facelift, brow lift, upper and lower eyelid lifts, laser skin resurfacing around mouth and eyes

with healing? Do you take medications that thin the blood? Also tell your surgeon about autoimmune conditions, such as rheumatoid arthritis, that may require you to take drugs that suppress your immune system, which could delay healing and make you susceptible to infection.

Are You a Nonsmoker?

Smoking is always a health risk. As mentioned earlier, it reduces blood flow to the cells and reduces the amount of oxygen released to the cells. There is evidence, however, that a deep-plane facelift is safer than the standard facelift for people who do smoke. With a deep-plane facelift, the tissue being moved is much thicker and has a much better blood supply. In addition, the surgeon is not applying tension to the skin, which in itself restricts blood flow.

Nevertheless, your doctor will want you to abstain from smoking for two weeks before surgery and for an additional two weeks throughout the healing process.

Undergoing a Deep-Plane Facelift

You will sleep throughout your surgery with the aid of anesthesia. Incision placement varies.

- The surgeon will make several small incisions along the hairline from the temple down to the top of the ear, along the natural creases in the skin in front of the ear (inside the ear for women), below the earlobe, and behind the ear.
- The full breadth of the drooping tissue to the level of the deep-plane tissue is incorporated into the facelift *flap*—this is the tissue that will be repositioned.
- The flap is gently lifted, positioned, and the deep fascia, the fibrous tissue that covers the muscles, is sutured to a stable area in front of the ear.
- The skin and soft tissue are redraped and the excess is trimmed.
- The skin is reattached and the incision closed using a combination of skin clips, removable sutures, and dissolvable sutures, according to your surgeon's preference.
- Also during the procedure, the surgeon will make a small incision under the chin in order to tighten the *platysma*, the neck muscle; then excess fat is suctioned away.

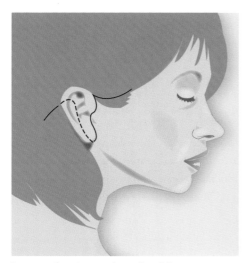
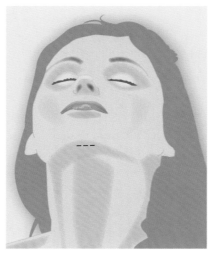

Incision for deep-plane facelifts

Incision for neck lift, which is part of a deep-plane lift

Drainage Tubes

Your surgeon may insert tubes in the incisions behind your ears to drain away excess fluid. These will be removed the day after surgery.

After Your Facelift

You will be taken to the recovery room and remain there about an hour, until the anesthesia wears off and you are able to walk about. You'll have a dressing wrapped under your chin and around the top of your head, leaving your face exposed. At this point, if your doctor approves and you have arranged for home care, you can be driven home. You'll still be tired and maybe a little groggy from the anesthesia.

Once at home, you'll need a caregiver, who can stay with you overnight and drive you to the surgeon's office the next day. You need to be surrounded by people who are supportive. You need to be free of distractions. At a minimum, a caregiver will accompany you home and stay with you for an hour or two.

The caregiver will see to it that you walk a bit that evening and that you take in plenty of fluids. Some doctors recommend the high-energy drink Gatorade.

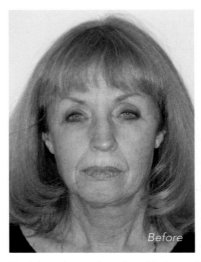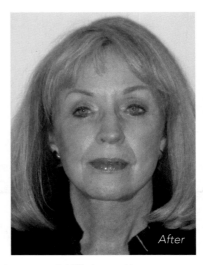

Revision deep-plane facelift, brow lift, lower eyelid lift, laser skin resurfacing around the eyes and mouth

More and more patients are choosing to stay with a professional caregiver at a nearby hotel or in a suite within the surgeon's clinic. These caregivers are specially trained to monitor your condition. He or she will make sure you don't exert yourself in any way, not even bending to pick something up.

Some facial cosmetic surgeons offer a private, clinic-operated retreat. Some patients stay overnight; four days is the norm. These settings offer patients a support network with access to a patient coordinator, the medical staff, and other patients past and present. You'll get continual feedback and reassurance that everything you're experiencing is normal, and immediate attention in the unlikely event of a complication.

Side Effects

Some side effects are milder with a deep-plane facelift than after a standard facelift. The symptoms listed below are normal and temporary. Even so, if your side effects seem unusual or they alarm you, do not hesitate to call your doctor's office right away. A "false alarm" is much better than ignoring a warning sign because you don't want to embarrass yourself or "bother" your doctor.

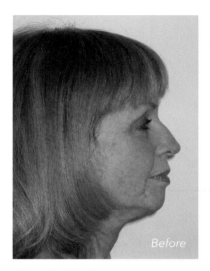
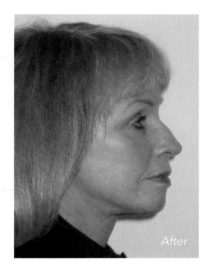

Before   *After*

Patient's side view

"*Today, facelift surgery is not painful, and bruising can be kept to a minimum. Patients can usually get back into their normal routines in about two weeks. However, complete healing takes longer.*"
—Neil A. Gordon, M.D.

Bruising and Redness

There is little or no bruising with a deep-plane facelift. If you have had lasering under the eyes, there will be some redness, which you can cover with concealer when appropriate. Some makeup experts suggest that using a green base under a skin-color concealer is the best way to cover the temporary redness after a laser treatment.

Swelling

The amount of swelling varies—full faces tend to swell more. By the third or fourth day after surgery, the swelling should be decreasing greatly. Within two weeks swelling is usually not readily apparent.

Seroma

Seroma, an accumulation of clear fluid, sometimes occurs behind the ear soon after a deep-plane facelift. Though it is seldom a cause for concern, you should notify your doctor. He or she might want to drain it as a precaution against infection.

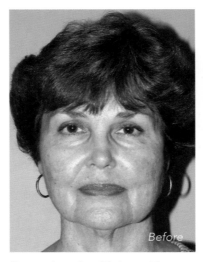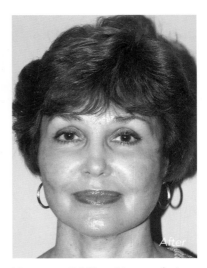

Before *After*

Deep-plane facelift, brow lift, upper and lower eyelid lifts, skin resurfacing around the eyes and mouth

Numbness

Numbness, too, is temporary and normal. With swelling there is a general numbness that disappears as the swelling goes down. Numbness around the ears and on the brow can last for several months.

Pain or Discomfort

Stiffness and tightness after a deep-plane facelift can be annoying and uncomfortable, but there is usually no pain. Since the deep-plane facelift is accomplished at a level that has minimal pain fibers, the majority of patients do not find the procedure painful, and use no pain medication. You'll have pain medication available, but if you're like most people who have had deep-plane facelifts you won't use it.

If you have severe pain, contact your doctor immediately. The pain could signify hematoma, infection, or another complication that needs prompt attention.

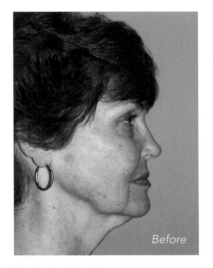 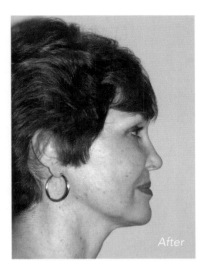

Before *After*

Patient's side view

Low Mood

The mild depression that sometimes follows cosmetic surgery can almost always be prevented. Low mood after surgery can be avoided if:

- Your expectations were realistic to begin with.
- You have listened to your doctor and educated yourself about what to expect and when to expect it.
- You have plenty of support from family and friends.
- You have planned well for your recovery by making arrangements for your usual responsibilities to be met and by preventing boredom with books, movies, visits from friends, and other pleasant but undemanding activities.
- You do everything your doctor has prescribed to speed healing.

Incision-Line Visibility

As the incisions heal, they will fade almost to invisibility. Eventually, only you and the surgeon will even know they're there. This may take several months. In the meantime, you can easily camouflage them with makeup.

There is no ear distortion with a deep-plane facelift. In fact, the procedure is often used to correct ear distortion from an earlier standard facelift.

Potential Complications

The greatest risk of complications comes from not following the surgeon's instructions. This means that complications can usually be prevented. Some patients are so aware of this that they are afraid to let their doctor know if something's wrong.

Do not be embarrassed or ashamed to contact your doctor immediately if you are concerned about a symptom. It doesn't matter if it's "your fault." What matters is that you get immediate medical attention if a complication does arise.

Hematoma

A hematoma is a collection or pool of blood outside a blood vessel. It is an uncommon complication after a facelift. However, if you do experience severe pain, a hematoma may be the cause. Get immediate medical attention to prevent healing problems.

Nerve Injury

There is a heightened risk of nerve damage with a deep-plane facelift if the surgeon is not highly skilled and experienced with the procedure. In experienced hands, injury to a branch of the facial nerve is exceedingly rare with deep-plane facelifts. The nerves are protected by a sheet of fascia that are not involved in the procedure. A surgeon who has done the procedure many times knows exactly where the nerves and protective fascia are located.

Infection

Infection is less likely with a deep-plane facelift than with a standard facelift because of the strong blood supply to the deeper tissues. In addition, antibiotics you take by mouth and that are given during surgery make infection extremely unusual.

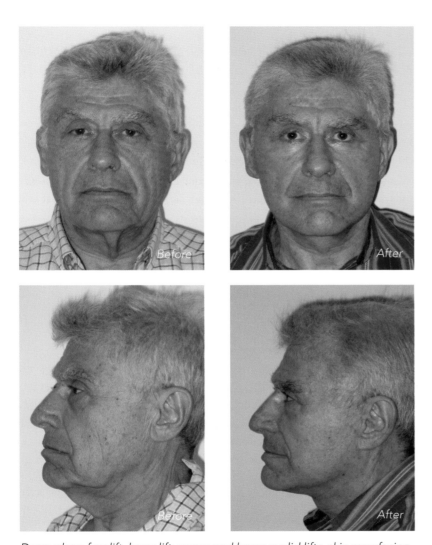

Deep-plane facelift, brow lift, upper and lower eyelid lifts, skin resurfacing around the eyes

Slow Healing

Smokers and patients with underlying health problems may heal more slowly than normal. Their progress will be steady, it will just take longer. Discuss any concerns about the rate of healing with your doctor.

When to Contact Your Surgeon

You should call your doctor's office any time you're concerned about a symptom. If you have pain, tenderness, inflammation, unusual swelling—anything that doesn't look right or doesn't feel right and isn't listed as a normal side effect—err on the side of caution and contact your doctor.

One of the things to consider when you're choosing a doctor is how well managed the office is. In a well-run office, if you call during office hours expressing alarm about a symptom, you will be connected with a nurse or physician right away or have your call returned within minutes. And since not all symptoms make themselves known during office hours, a well-managed practice will have given you instructions about after-hour emergencies.

Recovery

Recovery is similar to that for a standard facelift. For the first several days it's important to get plenty of rest, avoid any activity that raises your pulse or blood pressure, and keep your head above your heart—no bending over or heavy lifting. It's so automatic, when there's a tissue or a stray sock in the middle of the floor, to pick it up that you might have to keep reminding yourself how important it is to keep your head above your heart. A sudden rush of blood to the head could compromise the results of your surgery. Sleep with your head elevated, using a wedge-type pillow or raising your mattress at the top of the bed.

You can probably shower and wash your hair a day or two after surgery. Men can shave the day after surgery but should avoid the incision lines. You can gently brush your teeth the next day.

Sudden or jarring movements can damage the sutures, which is why driving a car is prohibited for a time. Driving usually is restricted for the first week after surgery.

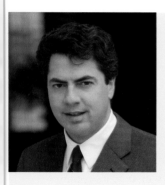

Neil A. Gordon, M.D.
Facial Plastic Surgeon
Greenwich, CT

What do you find most rewarding about your work? It is rewarding when patients trust me to perform cosmetic surgery on their faces and then appreciate what I have done and say that it exceeded their expectations. We provide more than just a surgical procedure. We offer an environment, in which we educate the patient, make them comfortable, and provide them privacy and pampering.

Describe the types of patients you see. What procedures are they seeking? The majority of patients I see are coming for facial rejuvenation. They range in age from thirty-five to eighty, with the most common age between late forties and sixty-five. They don't want to look different—they like their faces, but they want to reverse the signs of aging. They don't want look tired or as if they are frowning.

What has been one of the biggest, recent advances in the field of cosmetic surgery? One of the biggest changes has been our ability to perform facial rejuvenation through advances in facelifting techniques. The procedures we do today result in a more natural look; the procedures are also less invasive and longer lasting.

What procedures are you doing now that you didn't do five years ago? We are doing modifications of face lifting and brow lifting. As I mentioned, these are less invasive so the recovery is shorter and patients have less down time.

How have patients responded to these procedures? The response has been very positive. However, it's important that we educate our patients about the techniques and procedures we have available today. And just because a procedure is new and different, doesn't mean it's better for every patient. We want to make sure we choose the right procedures in order to meet the patient's goal.

What new developments are yet to come in facial cosmetic surgery? I think we'll see continued improvement in lasers and tissue fillers (for lines and wrinkles). I think one day we will use medical science to delay the signs of aging before they actually occur.

Describe one the most memorable patients you have seen recently. This would be a woman who came to me for revision work. Thirty-five percent of my patients come to me for revision procedures. This woman had already had two facelifts; her results were not optimal—a midface lift had resulted in her lower eyelids drooping. Given this experience, she was very fearful of having more surgery. But I was able to help her by first assuring her of the result I could give her and then delivering on that. She was quite pleased.

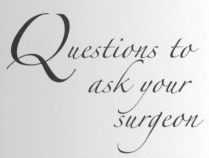

Questions to ask your surgeon

1. How many deep-plane facelifts have you performed?

2. Do I need a procedure such as a brow lift to compliment my facelift?

3. What should I do if I have concerns when the clinic is closed?

4. For how long after surgery will I need a caregiver?

5. When can I resume normal activities such as exercise?

6. Will I be able to wear glasses or contacts right away?

7. When will I be able to see the "finished product"?

Your doctor will advise you not to smoke and to avoid any medications that could thin the blood. Aspirin and food supplements (including essential fatty acid products such as fish oil) are among the many products that have blood-thinning effects. Your doctor will give you a complete list of drugs and over-the-counter products to avoid. He or she will recommend against alcohol to minimize bruising; it's also dangerous to mix alcohol with pain or sleep medications.

Good nutrition is a very important part of healing. Your doctor may prescribe an easily digested diet for a day or so after surgery. It is not uncommon to lose a few pounds after your procedure. Your doctor will council you on nutrition if weight loss is not desired. In addition, you should drink plenty of fluids.

Follow your doctor's instructions regarding cold compresses to reduce swelling, and topical products,such as Scar Guard or silicone gel, to help incisions heal properly. Your doctor will offer you other suggestions to aid in your aftercare program.

Returning to Work

With normal healing, you can probably go back to work within two weeks. If your job is physically demanding, talk to your doctor about specific activities you can and cannot undertake.

Going Out in Public

Wait a week or so before venturing out. If you still look a little puffy, you might want to delay your first public appearance a little longer. It's up to you and how self-conscious you might feel.

Exercising

After two to three weeks, you can ease into light exercise. Exercising in the first week could cause bleeding problems; light exercise in the next few weeks may create temporary swelling Take it slow at first, and stop if you notice any swelling.

Resuming Sexual Relations

Follow the same restrictions as for exercising. During the first two to three weeks, abrupt elevations in your heart rate or blood pressure can aggravate swelling and thus delay healing.

Direct sunlight is your skin's enemy. Incisions and lasered areas are especially vulnerable. Incision scars that are exposed to sunlight could become permanently darkened, in the first few months. Areas of skin that have been lasered could be more easily burned.

Even people who haven't had facial cosmetic surgery are cautioned to wear a hat outdoors and use sunscreen (applied at least half an hour before you go out) with SPF 15 at the very least. Those who ignore this advice will deal with sun-damaged skin at some point in the future. If you've had cosmetic surgery, you'll pay a higher and more immediate price. Why risk the investment of time and money you've made in your surgery by being careless about sun protection?

How Long Will a Deep-Plane Facelift Last?

As mentioned earlier, it's difficult to pinpoint the exact number of years a deep-plane lift will last. Proponents of the deep-plane lift believe this type of lift is longer-lasting than other lifts, because the deeper layer of tissues, which do not stretch, are lifted and do not sag as one ages. For example, if you have a deep-plane facelift at age 50 and it makes you look 35—fifteen years younger than your chronological age—then when you're 65 you'll most likely look 50.

Few people need to have a deep-plane lift refreshed. Those who do are probably candidates for a SMAS lift or a more limited deep-plane facelift.

Combining Facelifts with Other Procedures

It's common to combine a deep-plane facelift with other procedures such as a browlift, eyelid lift, and laser resurfacing to rejuvenate the facial skin. Research has shown that combining facial plastic surgery procedures doesn't affect safety or healing time. In fact, combined procedures are recommended in most people in order to create a balanced, natural and harmonious appearance. Two weeks after surgery and skin resurfacing, most patients find they need only to camouflage the lasered area with makeup.

CHAPTER SIX

The Midface Lift

6

The Midface Lift

The midface lift started gaining popularity in the 1990s. You may not be as aware of this facelift as you are of the standard lift. If you're like many people, you may not know which parts of the face make up the midface. Think of the midface as a triangle, formed by the outer corners of the eyes and the corners of the mouth. The midface does not include the areas below the jawline. For most of us, the midface is where we see some of the first signs of aging as the tissues in this area begin to sag. This starts to become noticeable in our thirties and continues as we get older.

What Is a Midface Lift?

As the name states, a midface lift affects the midface region. Sometimes called a cheek lift, this procedure lifts tissues and pulls them upward; a midface lift is effective in restoring the fat pads on the cheeks, producing a more "mounded," youthful cheek. This lift also diminishes the nasolabial fold more than the SMAS facelift does. The midface lift is sometimes called a "vertical lift," because it lifts the midface tissues vertically.

The midface lift does not affect the jowls or neck; nor does it involve the removal of loose skin, which is done with an SMAS facelift or a deep-plane lift. Accordingly, smaller incisions are used in the midface lift, making the procedure less invasive.

Are You a Candidate for a Midface Lift?

Do you look fatigued or sad, due to sagging in your midface area, when in fact you are happy and full of vigor? Do your deepening nasolabial folds or early jowls make you look older than you feel? If so, and you are otherwise healthy, you may be a good candidate for a midface lift. Individuals who choose midface lifts are often in their late thirties or forties and don't have much loose skin to be removed.

Undergoing a Midface Lift

Your surgeon may use twilight sedation or general anesthesia for your midface lift; he or she will discuss this with you. The procedure usually takes a few hours.

During a midface lift procedure, the surgeon repositions the cheek fat pads, pulling them up to their original positions, higher on the cheekbones. The fat pads are sutured into place to keep them from sliding downward again. As the fat pads are repositioned upward, the underlying facial muscles and skin are also elevated and tightened, diminishing the nasolabial folds. The overall result is a smoother, younger-looking contour. The surgeon may choose from several techniques for performing the midface lift. All procedures involve lifting the tissue on the cheeks.

Endoscopic Midface Lift

In this procedure, the surgeon may use an endoscope, a tiny fiber-optic lens attached to a camera, to perform a midface lift. Through the endoscope, the physician can view a television monitor in the operating room to see the subcutaneous tissues and is able to perform the surgery by manipulating the endoscope's tools externally. Advantages of endoscopic surgery include smaller incisions.

An endoscopic midface lift is commonly referred to as an *endoscopic subperiosteal lift*. The *periosteum* is a fibrous tissue that covers all bones, including the cheekbones. In this procedure, the surgeon goes below this fibrous tissue and lifts the tissues, resulting in a lift that delivers a younger-looking midface.

The surgeon has options on where to place incisions through which the midface tissues will be repositioned. Some surgeons make three to five short incisions in the hairline. Other surgeons make an incision through the lower eyelid, on the inside or outside. (When using a lower-eyelid incision, the surgeon can also trim away excess skin, even though the typical midface lift does not involve the removal of skin.) Yet other surgeons may gain access to the cheek tissues through an incision inside the mouth. Once the incisions are made, the surgeon can separate skin, muscle, and fat from bone and then lift the tissues,

"If you are thinking of having a facelift, do your homework. Read about the surgery and search the Internet. See more than one surgeon and learn about their experience and background. Talk to patients who have had procedures done by each surgeon."

—William Truswell, M.D.

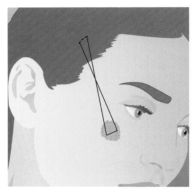

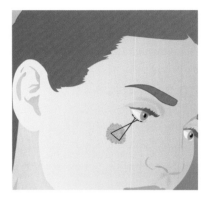

A surgeon may choose to perform a midface lift through incisions in the temple and lift the cheeks as shown above.

Some surgeons lift the midface through incisions on the inside of the lower eyelids.

anchoring them with sutures. The sutures may be anchored in the temple area or in the bone in the cheek area.

After Your Midface Lift

You should recover quicker from a midface lift than from a standard facelift. Swelling and bruising should diminish within a week, and you should be able to return to normal activities and to work within a week to ten days.

Side Effects

As with other facial surgeries, you can expect swelling in the cheeks and around the eyes, some minor bruising, and numbness. These are all temporary conditions.

Potential Complications

The biggest concern with a midface lift is putting too much tension on the lower eyelids and pulling them down too far. This happens rarely, and when it does it can be corrected. There is also a risk of nerve injury; however, this risk is minimized if you're in the

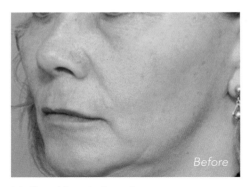

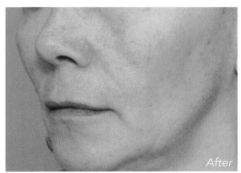

Midface lift with threads

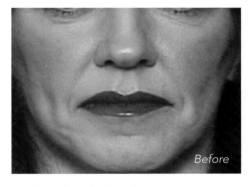

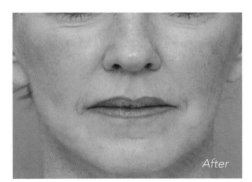

Midface lift with threads

Questions to ask your surgeon

1. Would a midface lift be the best option for me? Why?

2. Will the lift diminish my nasolabial fold?

3. Where will the surgery be performed?

4. What type of anesthesia is used?

5. How much discomfort can I expect?

6. How long will I need to take it easy?

7. When can I go back to work?

8. How soon can I drive after the surgery?

care of an experienced surgeon. Another possible complication is puckering at the corners of the eyes, if the incisions were made in the lower eyelids. This can be corrected in the doctor's office. Eyelid incisions can also produce eyelid shape changes.

How Long Will a Midface Lift Last?

A midface lift will generally last five to eight years. Lifestyle factors play a role in the length of time you maintain the results. Good nutrition, not smoking, and proper skin care will make the lift last longer.

> "The recovery process from facelift surgery is related to the complexity of the procedure and to the age and general health status of the patient. I always stress that there will be continued subtle improvement for several months after surgery."
>
> —Harrison C. Putman III, M.D.

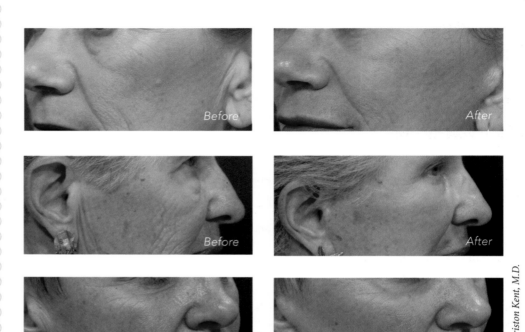

Courtesy of Kriston Kent, M.D.

Endoscopic midface lift

Other Approaches to Lifting the Midface

Other techniques are also being used to lift the midface. These involve suspension techniques—the *thread lift*, described in chapter 7, and a procedure known as an *Endotine midface lift*. For the Endotine lift, an incision is made in the temple area, above the ear, and the surgeon inserts a thin "leash," which has several tines (barbs) on the end of it. The device is pushed down into the cheek area, where the barbs attach to the cheek tissue, and the leash is pulled upward, lifting the cheek. The Endotine device is bioabsorbable, so it dissolves in seven to twelve months. By this time, the tissues have healed and reattached, so the cheek tissues stay suspended.

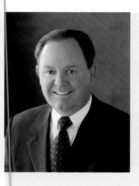

Harrison C. Putman III, M.D.
Facial Plastic Surgeon
Peoria, IL

What do you find most rewarding about your work? The primary reward is making a real difference in patients' quality of life, seeing them enjoy improved self-images. The artistry involved in cosmetic surgery is both challenging and rewarding. Each patient is unique, so it's important to assess the patient's situation, communicate a plan to that patient, and then execute it. I find this process very rewarding.

Describe the types of patients you see. What procedures are they seeking? The trend I see among patients is their interest in minimally invasive procedures that still accomplish a significant makeover. I call them "minimally invasive extreme makeovers." I am also seeing other trends, such as husbands and wives coming in together, wanting surgery at the same time. I'm also seeing mothers and daughters coming in together as well as siblings.

What has been one of the biggest changes in cosmetic surgery in recent years? Certainly we've seen the advancement of the more minimally invasive facelift. And of course, there are the injectable fillers. But aside from the surgical procedures, another interesting trend I've observed is that people are becoming more sophisticated as consumers. They learn about various cosmetic procedures from TV programs, so they know what they want. I still have patients who come in and say, "What do you think I need?" but more often than not they are telling me what they think they need. Patients are more astute about cosmetic surgery.

What procedures are you doing now that you didn't do five years ago? I'm doing more minimally invasive procedures, including some aesthetic procedures for skin improvement and skin tightening.

How have patients responded to these procedures? Patients respond favorably. That's why across the country we're seeing such an increase in patients who are seeking these minimally invasive treatments. They are thrilled with the injectable fillers; I use several of them, including Restylane and Radiesse, both of which I really like. I also inject a lot of Botox to diminish frown lines.

What new developments are yet to come in facial cosmetic surgery? I think we are going to see more developments in injectable filling agents, other forms of Botox, and devices for nonablative skin rejuvenation and skin tightening. For example, I am involved in an investigational study for a new radio frequency device that can tighten skin and produce some fat reduction. This will be a way to reshape the face and neck without surgery, but with noticeable improvements.

Describe one of the most memorable patients you've had recently. Rather than single out one patient, I would say the patients who have had the most notable impact are those who had several procedures performed or a combination of facial rejuvenation procedures. We were able to obtain some dramatic improvements; these results stemmed from good communication between me and the patient. It is so important that the patient and the surgeon have candid discussions about what the patient wants, what particular feature or features bother the patient the most, and what's appropriate.

CHAPTER SEVEN

The Thread Lift

7

The Thread Lift

*J*ust as we continually see new developments in other areas of modern medicine, new developments in cosmetic surgery continue to emerge. Facelift surgery has come a long way since the 1960s, when most facelifts were "skin only" procedures that produced that telltale "wind tunnel" look.

Many of the newer cosmetic surgery techniques are market driven by people who want to improve their appearance at earlier ages, and are not quite ready for a standard facelift. Enter the thread lift, a lift that is relatively noninvasive and requires less recovery time than the standard lift.

The thread lift was first developed by a Russian surgeon in the 1990s. The Food and Drug Administration approved the use of the threads for cosmetic surgery in 2004.

What Is a Thread Lift?

A *thread lift* is a procedure that lifts sagging areas of the face with barbed threads inserted under the facial skin, where they attach to underlying tissues. The surgeon softens contours of the face by gently pulling the threads upward and anchoring them into place in the temple area. An advantage to using the barbed threads is that they distribute the tension over the entire length of the thread rather than in one focal point with a suture. This produces a smoother, more natural look. The threads, made of clear polypropylene—a strong, lightweight plastic—have long been used for medical purposes, including heart surgeries.

How does a thread lift differ from a standard facelift? The thread lift is minimally invasive and does not involve the removal of loose skin. The thread lift accomplishes roughly 30–50 percent of what a traditional facelift does. (In addition to lifting the midface, the threads can also be used to lift the neck and the brow.)

You may have heard of thread lifts by other names, such as contour thread lift, cable thread lift, feather lift, suspended suture lift, or Aptos thread lift, named after a company that manufactures the threads.

A thread lift is not a replacement for a facelift but it can be used to pospone a facelift for a couple of years.

Are You a Candidate for a Thread Lift?

The best candidates for thread lifts are women and men in their late thirties to mid-forties who are in good health—physically and mentally—but who are showing early signs of aging. Other candidates for this procedure are those who, because of time constraints or budget, don't want to undergo a full facelift. The surgery is also popular among those who have had previous SMAS skin-only facelifts and want a little more lifting.

Who is *not* a good candidate for a thread lift? The thread lift is not considered a good option for individuals with a great deal of loose facial or neck skin since the procedure does not involve the excision, or trimming away, of any skin. The procedure only lifts sagging skin. Others who may not be good candidates are those with very thin, fragile skin or those who have heavy faces.

An important note: Even though the thread lift is applauded by many as a quicker and easier cosmetic procedure, remember it is still surgery. The procedure requires some recovery time, and the risk for complications is real, making it important to choose a surgeon who is experienced in performing the procedure.

Undergoing a Thread Lift

If you undergo a thread lift, you'll probably be fully awake for the procedure, which takes about an hour. You may be given an oral sedative to help you relax; you'll receive local anesthesia injections that contain lidocaine, a commonly used anesthetic, and epinephrine, which constricts blood vessels and helps prevent bleeding. Your face will be swabbed with an antiseptic solution to kill surface bacteria, and the surgeon will put markings on your face to guide him or her in inserting the threads.

To lift the midface, the surgeon first makes a tiny incision in the hairline near the ear. Through this incision, the surgeon will guide a needle under the skin down toward the jowl

> "*T*hread lifts may be used to lift the cheeks, the jowls, or the brow. These can all be lifted at once, or they may be performed as separate procedures."
>
> —William Truswell, M.D.

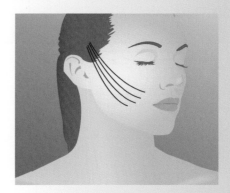

Thread placement for cable thread lift for the face

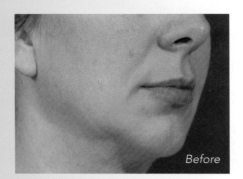

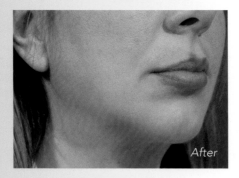

Cable thread lift, lifting the jowls

and chin. The needle carries the barbed thread, which catches on the underlying tissues. The surgeon gently pulls the threads upward, giving lift to the sagging skin. The surgeon may use between sixteen and twenty threads, depending on which parts of the face are being lifted. For example, two threads are used on each side of the face for the midface, four threads for each cheek, and four threads on each side of the neck. If the eyebrows are being lifted, it will require two threads on each side.

Once the thread is in place, the needle is removed and the threads are cut and anchored in the temple area. Because polypropylene threads are clear, they don't show through the skin. The tension in the threads can be adjusted, so, for example, if the surgeon determines the skin was lifted too much, the threads can be relaxed. In fact, the threads can be removed altogether if the patient so desires, or additional threads can be added as needed.

After the procedure is completed, the surgeon may apply a light tape to your face, along the course of the underlying threads. You'll be asked to wear this tape for several days; the tape helps stabilize the cheeks and serves to remind you to not touch your face and possibly dislodge a thread while the tissues are healing. Some surgeons may use a light compression bandage, such as an Ace bandage, rather than the tape, to remind patients not to rub their faces.

After Your Thread Lift

Although the recovery from a thread lift is much easier than from a traditional facelift, your face will be sore and you'll need to take it easy for seven days. Your surgeon will probably instruct you to apply cold cloths to your face over the next twenty-four to forty-eight hours. Wet a cloth in ice water and wring it out. This will help control soreness and swelling. Avoid using ice packs—if used too long, the ice could injure your skin; also, the weight of ice could dislodge the threads.

In fact, you will want to avoid any pressure on your face for the next thirty days. Do not rub, scrub, or massage your face in any way. You'll be asked to use a small or horseshoe-shaped pillow for three weeks so that you don't roll over while sleeping and put pressure on the threads.

You should minimize your facial movements for two weeks to avoid snapping a suture. This means avoid excessive talking or making animated facial expressions. Similarly, avoid eating foods, such as apples, that place greater stress on your facial muscles. Men are asked to not shave for one week and then to shave lightly with upward strokes for an additional two weeks in order not to disturb the threads.

Side Effects

The general side effects that accompany a thread lift are similar to the side effects you would experience with other types of facial cosmetic surgery. These include swelling, bruising, numbness, and soreness. There are also other side effects unique to thread lifts:

- Temporary overcorrection. It may appear that the face has been lifted too much. However, this effect settles within the first few days after the procedure.
- Skin "bunching." It's usual to have some skin "bunching" or "pleating" near the incision site, where the threads are pulled and anchored. This is to be expected and typically settles in two to six weeks.
- Skin irregularities. You may develop wrinkles or irregularities in the skin along the path of the threads. These will diminish in the days ahead. If they don't, the surgeon may smooth the skin manually.
- Feeling threads with facial movements.

Potential Complications

The rate of complications with thread lifts has been low, and the risk is decreased if you are in the hands of a skilled, experienced surgeon. However, potential complications are like those in other types of cosmetic surgery, including infection, hematoma, and seroma. There are also risks of other complications:

- Asymmetry. One side of the face may not match the other side. If this should occur, the threads can be adjusted as needed.
- Thread breakage. A thread may break and poke out through the skin. If this occurs, the thread may come out by itself or your surgeon may need to remove it. In some cases, the thread may not be retrievable and will remain in the face; however, the remaining thread is usually not cause for concern.
- Thread exposure. There is a possibility that the thread can be felt through the skin. If this happens, the thread can be

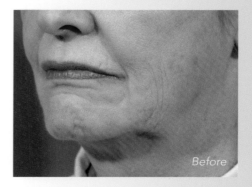

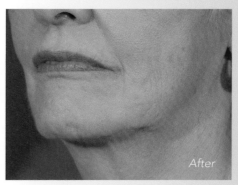

Facelift with threads

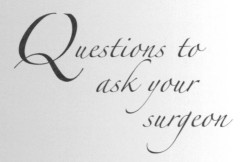

Questions to ask your surgeon

1. Is a thread lift the right procedure for me?

2. What parts of my face can be treated with a thread lift?

3. How long might the results last?

4. What type of anesthesia do you use when performing a thread lift?

5. Have your patients experienced complications? If so, what were they, and how did you treat them?

6. How long will I be off work?

7. When can I resume rigorous exercise?

removed. In some cases, the thread softens and does not require removal.

- Pain at thread site.

How Long Will a Thread Lift Last?

Although you'll see immediate results, the full effect of the thread lift will not be visible until three to six months later. By that time, your natural collagen will have formed around the threads, helping to maintain the lifting effect. How long can you expect the thread lift to last? As with other cosmetic surgeries, the length of time the procedure lasts varies among individuals. Generally, the effects of a thread lift will last from months to years, depending on where you are in the aging process. Some patients return to their surgeons two to three year later for a longer-lasting procedure.

Combining Thread Lifts with Other Procedures

It is possible to have other cosmetic procedures performed along with the thread lift. Some individuals choose to have a brow lift or a neck lift, also performed with threads, at the time of their thread lift. You can also receive Botox injections or undergo skin rejuvenation treatment, including chemical peels or laser resurfacing (see chapter 11), at the same time as the thread lift procedure.

Does a thread lift prevent you from having other facial cosmetic surgery in the future? No. You can still undergo a standard facelift later if you choose. If you should do so, the threads will likely be left in place. Interestingly, some cosmetic surgeons are using threads as part of a standard facelift procedure, to help maintain the lift to the midface.

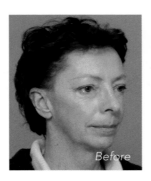
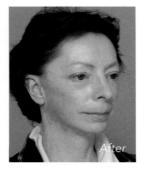

Before   After

Since no skin is removed during a thread lift, the surgeon deliberately "overcorrects" when lifting the skin. This creates a temporary "bunching" of skin under the ear; this skin will smooth out in one to two weeks.

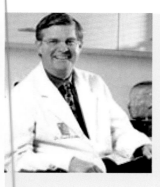

David A. F. Ellis, M.D.
Facial Plastic Surgeon
Toronto, Canada

What do you find most rewarding about your work? What I find totally rewarding is that I make patients happy. We expect good results in plastic surgery and we get them. Our patients are not suffering from serious diseases, so we have a pleasant emotional environment. I also find the work challenging; we are constantly seeing new developments in cosmetic surgery.

Describe the types of patients you see. What procedures are they seeking? Today, more patients are interested in refreshing their faces by adding volume. As we age, some of the tissues that plump up the face shrink away. In the past, we focused on eliminating the sag in the face, which means we've done facelifts and thread lifts; now, in addition to those procedures, we are concentrating on volume. So, it's a balance between elevating, lifting, and restoring volume to the midface.

What has been one of the biggest changes in cosmetic surgery in recent years? The way I practiced facial plastic surgery twenty-five years ago is completely different from what I do today. We now have new, less invasive techniques; the procedures produce good results and patients heal more quickly.

What procedures are you doing now that you didn't do five years ago? It would be the large volume soft tissue filler. In Canada, we have approval to use a permanent injectable implant, called Bio-Alcamid. Since it is a large volume filler, I can inject twenty to thirty cubic centimeters at a time. After it's injected, the surgeon smoothes the material manually. It's also reversible—if I inject too much in an area, I can draw it out. Before using this filler, I was using a lot more fat for reimplantation. This filler is not yet available in the United States, but likely will be within a few years. Also, I'm doing a lot of thread lifts, which I was not doing five years ago.

How have patients responded to these procedures? Patients love the permanent filler, and there are really very few complications with the procedure. My patients like the thread lifts, too. We expect patients to get two to three years of improvement with the thread lifts. Of course, patients would like them to last longer, but the improvement is good and there's very little downtime.

What new developments are yet to come in facial cosmetic surgery? I think we'll see new technology in skin care—treatments to slow aging on the surface of the skin. Heretofore, we've focused on the tissues under the skin.

Describe one of the most memorable patients you've had recently. I remember a woman who was not really overweight, but she had a lot of fat on her face and she had no neckline. Her jaw went right down into her neck without a defining neckline. I performed a brow lift and facelift with heavy liposuction. Actually, I recontoured her whole face. She was so pleased because it was the first time in her life she had ever had a jawline.

CHAPTER EIGHT

The Mini Facelift

8

The Mini Facelift

As you know by now, there are a variety of ways to lift the face. You've heard about the standard SMAS lift, the deep-plane lift, the midface lift, and the thread lift. There is yet another lift being offered by cosmetic surgeons: the "mini" lift. It is often thought to be a facelift for the busy person who wants to rejuvenate his or her face, but doesn't want to take much time to recuperate. In fact, recovery time from a mini facelift is shorter than recovery from a standard facelift. Typically, the mini facelift costs less than the standard facelift.

What Is a Mini Facelift?

A mini facelift is a procedure that tightens loose skin on the face and neck. Because it typically uses smaller incisions, this lift is a less invasive procedure than a standard facelift. However, it's important to be aware that many types of mini facelifts are being marketed today, and they are not all the same procedure. Some procedures offer only minimal results that are not long lasting—only skin is tightened. Other mini lifts elevate the SMAS, providing a "deeper" lift that will last several years.

You'll hear the mini facelift being referred to by many names, including the "short scar lift," the "weekend lift," or the "S-lift," so called because of the shape of the incision. If a mini lift interests you, make sure you clearly understand what the procedure you're inquiring about will accomplish.

Are You a Candidate for a Mini Lift?

The ideal age for a mini lift candidate depends on the complexity of the lift itself. If the lift is minimal and does not elevate the underlying tissues of the face, the best candidates are people in their thirties or forties, since they don't have much loose tissue.

For older persons, who do have lax skin in the face or neck, a mini facelift can produce results if it also lifts the SMAS layer. A mini lift is also an option for persons who have had a standard facelift and now want a touch-up procedure.

Expectations are important when determining whether you are a candidate for a mini lift. If you are considering a mini lift, it is important to understand that facial changes need to match to the procedure. In other words, if no other procedures are done in combination with the mini lift, the result might be an unbalanced appearance.

Undergoing a Mini Facelift

For a mini facelift, you may receive any type of anethesia. Some surgeons are performing these procedures with local anesthesia combined with an oral sedative.

The type of incision the surgeon uses can vary. Some surgeons will use an incision similar to that used in a standard facelift, only shorter. The incision may begin in front of the ear and go down in front of the ear canal before curving around the earlobe and going behind the ear. This incision is made on both sides of the head. Some surgeons will keep the incision just inside the ear canal so that no scar shows in the sideburn area.

Some mini lifts remove loose skin only; other surgeons perform mini lifts that also elevate and reposition the SMAS layer. Incisions are closed with fine sutures. Liposuction may also be performed to remove fat from the jowl area. The procedure takes about sixty to ninety minutes.

After Your Mini Facelift

The type of bandage used will vary among surgeons. You may have an elastic bandage wrapped under your chin and around the top of your head; usually, you're asked to wear this for the first twenty-four hours after surgery.

If you had twilight sedation, you may feel slightly groggy. If you received only a local anesthetic with an oral sedative, you may not feel groggy, but still should not drive. Your caregiver should drive you home.

You will minimize swelling by sleeping with your head elevated on several pillows. In most cases, you can wear makeup immediately following the procedure.

"Follow your surgeon's postoperative instructions carefully. You'll need to take it easy for the first few days after your procedure. You'll be told when you may return to normal activities. More strenuous activities will require a little more time."

—Jon Mendelsohn, M.D.

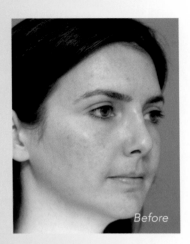

Before

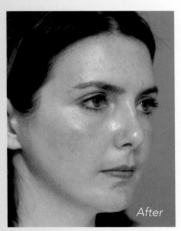

After

Mini facelift

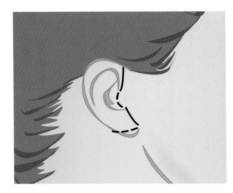

For a woman, the mini lift incision may be partially inside the ear.

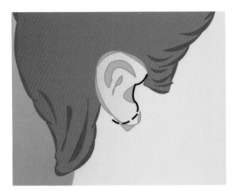

For a man, the mini lift incision needs to be outside the ear canal to avoid pulling the beard into the ear canal.

Recovery with this procedure is relatively quick. Most individuals can resume light activities, including going back to work, within the first week and can resume most other activities after three weeks. Your sutures will be removed within five to seven days, and any visible scars should become almost imperceptible over time.

Side Effects and Potential Complications

The side effects of a mini facelift are fewer than in a standard facelift. The mini facelift produces minimal bruising, which peaks at two days and then diminishes. Swelling is also minimal.

The risk of complications with a mini facelift is similar to that of other facelifts. There is a very small risk of postoperative bleeding, infection, nerve damage, or scarring. In some patients, the earlobe might become numb, but this should be temporary.

How Long Will a Mini Facelift Last?

The length of time a mini facelift will last depends on the type of mini facelift you have, your genes, the amount of sun damage you incur, and your lifestyle habits. For many people, a mini facelift can last between five and seven years.

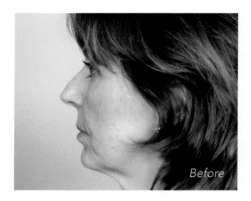
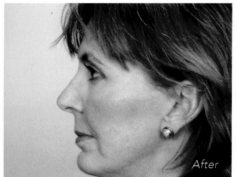
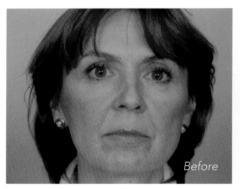
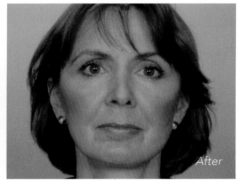

Mini facelift, chin augmentation, nose reshaping

Questions to ask your surgeon

1. Am I a candidate for a mini lift?

2. What does the mini lift you perform involve?

3. Does your mini lift elevate the SMAS layer?

4. What are the advantages and disadvantages of a mini lift?

5. What kind of anesthesia is used?

6. How soon can I return to work?

7. How will a mini lift affect future cosmetic surgeries?

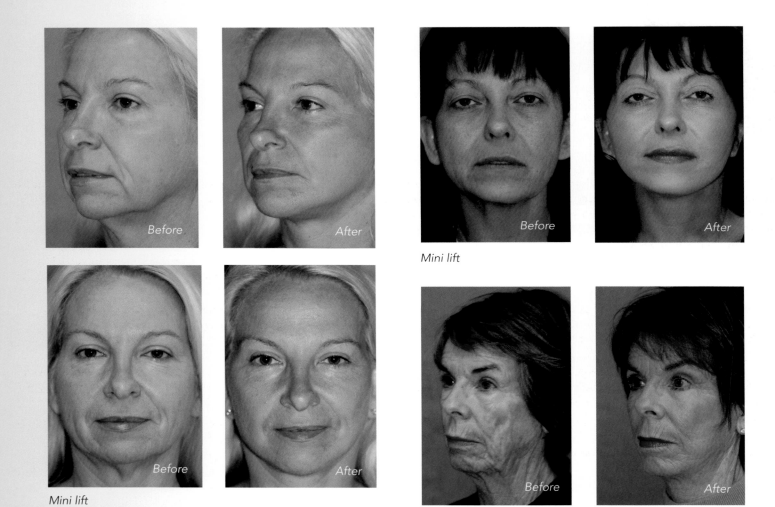

Mini lift

Mini lift

Mini lift

Mini lift

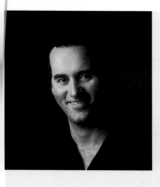

Jon Mendelsohn, M.D.
Facial Plastic Surgeon
Cincinnati, OH

What do you find most rewarding about your work? Probably one of the most rewarding things for me is being part of changing people's lives. No matter how insignificant a cosmetic surgery procedure may seem to others, I see my patients leaving happy and with increased confidence and self-esteem as a result of a better appearance. And, because they're happier, they have better relationships with family, friends, and coworkers. They just feel better about themselves.

Describe the types of patients you see. What procedures are they seeking? Typically, I see happy, healthy patients, most of whom are women in the baby-boomer age bracket. They want to look as good as they feel; they usually feel that their faces look tired and they want to look more refreshed. So rather than wait until they are in their sixties, patients who are forty-five or fifty are coming in. They are looking for more subtle, natural-looking results. They don't want to make drastic changes at one point in their lives; they want to maintain their appearance throughout their lives.

What has been one of the biggest changes in cosmetic surgery in recent years? Without question, it's the ability to provide full facial rejuvenation in a shorter period of time, less invasively, and without the need for anesthesia. Certainly, many of the advances in fillers, such as the hyaluronic acid (Restylane) in particular and Botox have made a really big difference in achieving what patients are asking for. They are seeking treatments that are both quick and that have more lasting results.

What procedures are you doing now that you didn't do five years ago? I am doing a mini facelift differently from the way I did it five years ago. Now I do this lift with local sedation—no other anesthesia. And this is not a skin-only procedure. We are lifting the SMAS layer and removing the excess skin much as we would in a standard facelift. The mini lift improves the jawline and the neck area.

How have patients responded to these procedures? Patients have responded well. In fact, we have doubled the number of mini facelifts we're doing annually. We make shorter incisions, and we make the incisions inside the ear canal rather than in front of the ear. Patients like not having the scar in front of the ear. The procedure takes only about an hour.

What new developments are yet to come in facial cosmetic surgery? I think enhancing volume in the face is going to be important. Patients who are aging lose volume in their face, and facial rejuvenation is not always about lifting the tissues surgically; it's also about adding volume. I think we'll see the use of injectables for this. I think we'll also have improvements in laser technology; we'll also see more long-lasting products, such as Botox.

Describe one of the most memorable patients you've had recently. A woman came for a rhinoplasty—a nose job, a facelift, and eyelid surgery. She was just thrilled. It changed her life. Then, she sent one of her daughters in for rhinoplasty, and later sent another daughter for the same procedure. Soon after that, the woman's husband came in; he had a facelift and an eyelid lift. It was extremely rewarding to know that the woman's surgery affected her life so positively that she wanted her family members to have the same experience. There was nothing unusual about the surgeries really, but it was a little unusual that we ended up seeing so many members of one family.

CHAPTER NINE

Lip Augmentation and Facial Implants

9

Lip Augmentation and Facial Implants

Of all facial cosmetic procedures, facelifts seem to get the most press coverage. We see people getting facelifts on makeover television shows, and celebrities getting facelifts often makes headlines. However, two other procedures that you may not have heard as much about can also transform the face. These procedures are lip augmentation and facial implants.

Both facial implants and lip augmentation can be used to restore balance to your features and freshen your appearance. Let's first take a closer look at lip augmentation.

What Is a Lip Augmentation?

As we enter our late thirties, our lips begin to shrink slightly. They become thinner and paler as we age. Women tend to form vertical lines in the skin above the lip.

Lip augmentation is a procedure in which the lips are made fuller and smoother by the insertion of an implant or implant materials. An augmentation may include the entire lip or may be used only on the borders of the lips. In some cases, the augmentation may smooth fine wrinkles around the lips.

There are several types of implant materials. Implants may be injectable fillers, which are temporary, or they may be made of solid material, which are permanent.

Injectable Fillers

Injectable fillers are inserted into the lips with a fine needle. Today, some of the most commonly used fillers contain hyaluronic acid, a substance found naturally in our skin that helps maintain volume and moisture. Since injectable fillers are temporary, the procedure will need to be repeated in the months ahead. Brand names of commonly used hyaluronic acid products include Restylane, Perlane, and Hylaform.

Another filler, collagen, has been used as a soft tissue filler for years. It is made from cow or pig collagen, which is similar to human collagen. However, collagen can cause allergic reactions, so a skin test is required before it can be injected. A newer form of collagen, made from human collagen, does not require a pretest. Collagen brand names are CosmoDerm and CosmoPlast.

Solid Implants

The solid implant material used for lip augmentation is made of a soft, moldable rubber. This synthetic material comes in strips or threads that can be trimmed and shaped according to the needs of the patient. You may hear your surgeon refer to commonly used brands such as Gore-Tex, Advanta, SoftForm, and UltraSoft. Other substances can also be used for lip implants, including one's own fat tissue, which is harvested through a "mini-liposuction" procedure. Differences in implant material can affect the length of time the implant lasts, as well as potential side effects, such as lumps or asymmetries.

Lip Augmentation Materials	Injectable Lip Implants
Restylane	Gore-Tex
Hylaform	Advanta
Perlane	SoftForm
Radiesse	UltraSoft
CosmoDerm	AlloDerm
Artecoll	dermis grafts
bovine collagen	tendon grafts
Isolagen	fascia grafts

Are You a Candidate for a Lip Augmentation?

As required for all cosmetic surgery procedures, you should be in general good health. Your teeth should be clean and your gums healthy. Any dental work, including teeth cleaning, should be done well in advance of a lip augmentation procedure. Why? It's possible that dental work could release bacteria, which may increase the risk of infection after lip augmentation.

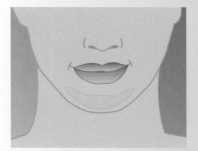

Frontal view of chin implant placement

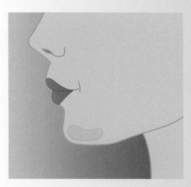

Side view of chin implant placement

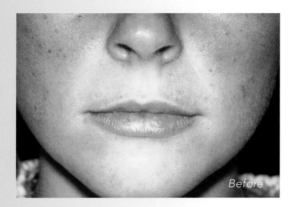

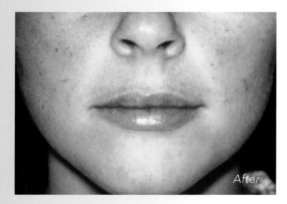

Upper lip enhancement

Individuals who may *not* be good candidates are those with disorders involving collagen (their own) or connective tissue, including lupus or scleroderma, or raised scars. Similarly, you may be advised not to undergo lip augmentation if you have uncontrolled diabetes or allergies to anesthetics. To prevent cold sores and other virus-related outbreaks, antiviral medications are given for all procedures.

Undergoing a Lip Augmentation

Most lip augmentations are performed in the cosmetic surgeon's office. If you're anxious, you may be offered a mild sedative to help you relax. Your lips and surrounding skin will be wiped with an antiseptic solution, and you will be given a local anesthetic. If you're undergoing a lip augmentation with the use of injectables, the surgeon will perform a series of injections with a very fine needle. It may require twelve to sixteen injections.

If your surgeon is inserting an implant material, the material is pulled, like a thread, through the lips. To accomplish this, the surgeon makes a tiny incision at the corner of each lip to be enhanced. Then, with a special threading device, the implant is pulled through the lip. The ends are trimmed and rounded and the tiny incision is closed with a single suture. This procedure may be done with anesthesia. The incisions will leave minimal to no visible scars.

If you are having your own fat injected into your lips, the fat is often taken from the abdomen. Once collected, the fat is placed in a centrifuge and spun to separate fat tissue from liquids. The surgeon then draws the fat into a syringe and injects it into the lips.

After a Lip Augmentation

Whether you've had your lips augmented with a temporary injectable or a permanent filler, you will leave the surgeon's office with immediate results—your lips will appear fuller. Of course, some of that fullness will be attributed to swelling, which will subside within a few days.

Because the nerves and muscles in your lips are affected, your lips may feel unusual for a few days. Such activities as drinking, eating, and speaking may be affected for a few days.

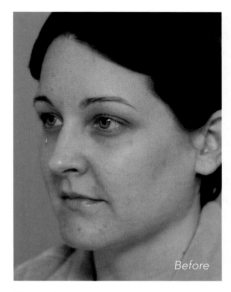
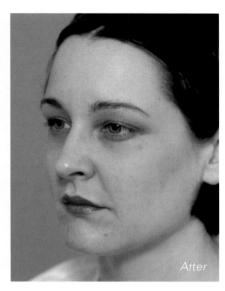

Before

After

Upper lip enhancement

You should be able to return to regular activities the day after the procedure. If you have had any type of sedation, be sure you have arranged to be driven home.

Side Effects

Swelling is the most common side effect after a lip augmentation. This swelling may last as long as a couple of weeks. Other side effects include numbness, dry lips, mild discomfort, lip asymmetries, and redness. Your surgeon may prescribe antibiotics to help prevent infection.

If you have had lip implants, you may initially have more swelling than that caused by injectables; you may also have some bruising. As the anesthetic wears off, you may find your lips sensitive to pressure for several days. Accordingly, you may wish to choose soft foods for the first few days.

Your surgeon will also instruct you to avoid any exaggerated movement with your lips—big yawns, broad smiles, and laughter. Such movements could cause the implant

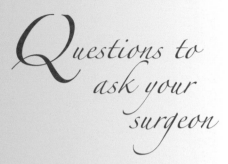

Questions to ask your surgeon

1. Should I have augmentation with an injectable filler or an implant?

2. How long will an injectable filler last?

3. What kind of anesthetic will you use? Will I feel groggy?

4. How much discomfort do patients typically have after the procedure?

5. How soon can I resume routine activities? Strenuous activities?

6. May I see before-and-after photos of your patients?

material to shift before it has settled into place. Ask your surgeon how soon you can wear lipstick. However, because your lips will be sensitive to pressure, you may wish to wait several days before applying lipstick.

Potential Complications

If you had lip augmentation with implants, there is a slight risk of the implant material migrating—shifting out of place. This would create a lumpy or asymmetrical look. Call your surgeon if this occurs.

In some cases, lip implant material becomes palpable, meaning you can feel it with your fingers. This is not normal, and you should consult your surgeon if it should occur. The newer implant materials on the market make such an occurrence less likely.

How Long Will a Lip Augmentation Last?

The length of time a lip augmentation lasts varies among individuals and depends on the type of material used. Solid implants are permanent. The temporary fillers, such as hyaluronic acid, will usually last three to nine months. Collagen fillers will last about three to four months. You'll notice a difference in the fullness of you lips as these materials are gradually reabsorbed by your body. One of the benefits of the temporary fillers is being able to see how you like the look of your augmented lips before choosing to have them augmented with a longer-lasting material.

What Are Facial Implants?

A facial implant is a medical-grade rubberlike or plastic device that is placed under the skin to augment a facial feature. The most commonly used implants are chin implants and cheek implants. They come in a wide range of sizes and styles, and are customized for the patient. Facial implants may be performed as a single procedure or can be done in combination with a facelift or other procedures.

Chin Implants

Chin augmentation, called *mentoplasty*, increases the projection of the chin. It is used to bring a receding chin into balance with the rest of the face. A receding chin can be perceived as a sign of weakness in both men and women; men often choose chin implants because a more prominent chin is also considered more masculine. Similarly, a weak chin can make the nose look larger than it is. Some patients who go to cosmetic surgeons inquiring about a rhinoplasty—a nose job—really need only a chin implant. When performed in combination with a facelift, the chin implant provides an extension of the chin, helping to create a more defined jawline.

You may think that a chin implant would affect only the appearance of your profile. But, interestingly, a chin implant also brings greater balance and symmetry to the frontal view of the face. How much projection should a chin implant create? This is a matter you can discuss with your surgeon; he or she will help you decide what size implant is appropriate. Current implants appear even more natural than those of the past because shapes now available subtly enhance the whole chin region.

Cheek Implants

Cheek implants, though not used as frequently as chin implants, can reduce a hollow or sunken look in your cheeks and can also correct underdeveloped cheekbones; the implants add fullness and lift to the cheeks, producing a healthier, more youthful look, especially for those with long faces.

Are You a Candidate for a Facial Implant?

If you are in overall good health, and have a weak chin or feel your cheeks are sunken, you may be a good candidate for a facial implant. During a consultation, a cosmetic surgeon will do a skeletal analysis of the bone structure of your face, noting any deficiencies in the cheeks or chin. One of the key features the surgeon looks for is facial symmetry. He or she will determine whether your face is balanced by comparing three regions of your face—the brow, the midface, and the chin and neck. Deficiencies are common and can be significantly improved with implants.

Facial implants are used for all ages, young and old alike. However, some patients find the aging process has especially made them good candidates for facial implants. It's common for the cheeks to become sunken and for the chin to get weaker and smaller as we age; bone is partially absorbed, causing a loss of contour and volume along the jawline and in the chin. This deficiency will be more apparent if you have had dental extractions in your

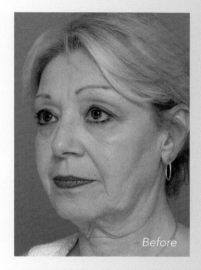
Before

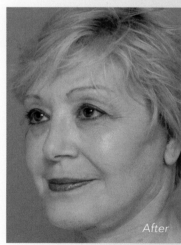
After

Chin implant and standard facelift

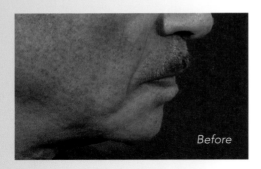

Before

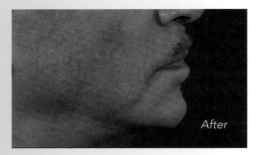

After

Chin implant

lower jaw. Losses in soft tissue and sagging of facial tissue also contribute to flattening of the cheekbone and loss of chin projection.

Undergoing a Chin or Cheek Implant

As you consult with your doctor prior to scheduling any surgery, make sure you tell him or her your medical history, including dental or gum problems. Also ask your doctor whether you will need someone to drive you to and from the surgery, and discuss any medications you are taking, such as aspirin, which increases the risk of bleeding during your surgery. On the day of the surgery, wear a loose-fitting top that does not have to be pulled over your head.

A facial implant procedure is normally done on an outpatient basis. Either a local or general anesthesia is administered, depending on your needs and the other procedures you are having.

For a chin implant, the incision is made inside the mouth, along the lower lip, or in the outer skin just under the chin. Once the necessary incisions are made, a pocket is formed and the implant is inserted. The surgeon then closes the incision. Your chin will be taped to minimize swelling. Most facial implant surgeries take from thirty minutes to an hour.

The procedure for a cheek implant is essentially the same as that for a chin implant. For a cheek implant, the incision can be made inside the upper lip or in the lower eyelid.

If a chin or cheek implant is being done in conjunction with a facelift, the implant is inserted through an incision already made for the facelift.

After a Facial Implant

Recovery from chin or cheek surgery is typically swift, with most swelling subsiding within a day or two and a return to work within the next five to seven days for most patients. For the next several weeks, you will want to avoid any activities that could result in your face being bumped.

Any sutures inside your mouth will dissolve in about ten days and will not require removal. You may also have dissolvable sutures under your chin; if not, the sutures will be removed in four to seven days.

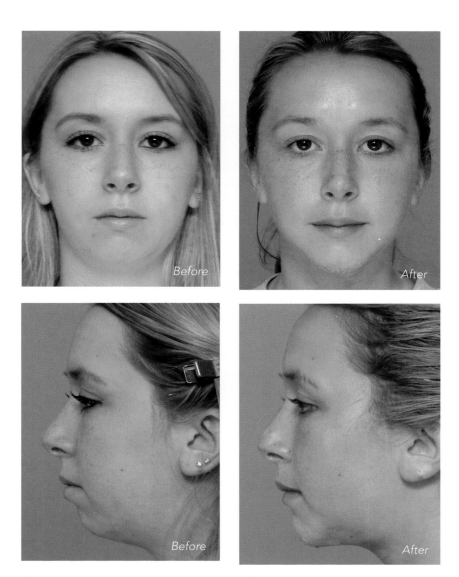

The chin implant also adds balance to the frontal view of the face.

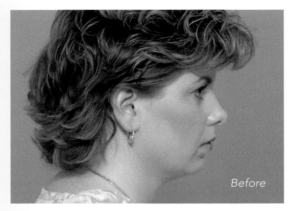
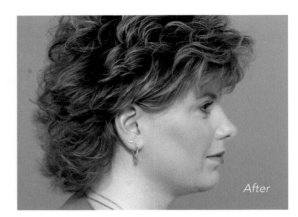

Before

After

Chin implant

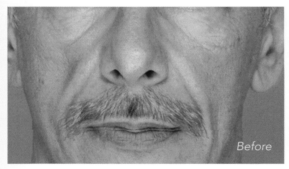
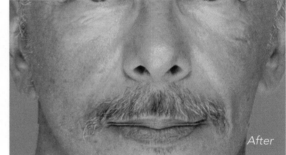

Before

After

Cheek implant and facelift

Side Effects

After a facial implant, you can expect facial swelling, which, in most cases, will be gone within several days to a week. Usually there is little or no bruising with facial implant surgery. With either a chin or cheek implant, you may have some tenderness or soreness for the next several days. It is common for numbness to occur in the chin region for about three months.

Potential Complications

There are few complications associated with facial implants. Asymmetry, in which the features on one side of the face do not match those on the other side, can occur, but this is uncommon. If this should happen, it is generally in the cheekbones and can be corrected by adjusting the implants. There is also a risk of the implant shifting, but in most cases only if it was placed incorrectly; a follow-up procedure can correct the problem.

Infection is rare, but if it should occur, an implant will extrude. Call your doctor if you develop a fever of 100 degrees or higher since such a symptom may be an indication of infection. Also call your surgeon if you experience abnormal pain, swelling, or any discharge at the site of the incision. Permanent numbness is rare.

How Long Will a Facial Implant Last?

Whether you have had a chin implant or a cheek implant, you should not have to have the procedure repeated later in life. Its effectiveness should not diminish, because the implant material and position does not change. The result is permanent, unless you have the implant removed.

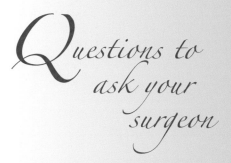

Questions to ask your surgeon

1. Where will you make incisions?

2. What kind of anesthetic will I receive?

3. Will I need pain medication afterward?

4. Is the implant permanent?

5. How will a chin implant affect the look of my nose?

6. When can I resume normal activities?

7. Will I have numbness?

CHAPTER TEN

Eyelid Lifts and Brow Lifts

10

Eyelid Lifts and Brow Lifts

Clearly, the eyes are one of the primary features of the face, and when the tissues around the eyes begin to age, our appearance is affected. As we grow older, the skin and muscle in our upper eyelids begin to thicken and sag. The lid may drape over the eye in varying degrees, distorting the shape of our eyes, making us look older and tired. Similarly, the lower lids may appear puffy—also the result of sagging skin and muscle and fat bulges. Actually, it's normal to have fat around the eyes—it protects them from injury. But as we age, the tissues around the fat sag, and the fat starts to protrude through that tissue, resulting in puffiness—a look that says, "I didn't get enough sleep last night."

The forehead ages as well, developing lines and drooping brows which contribute to partially covering our eyes. If you feel your appearance is affected by the effects of aging around your eyes, you may benefit from an eyelid lift or a brow lift. Often, cosmetic surgeons will recommend a combination of both in order to achieve the optimum results.

What Is an Eyelid Lift?

In performing an eyelid lift, called a *blepharoplasty*, the surgeon lifts the lids by removing sagging eyelid tissues. This procedure can be performed on both the upper and lower eyelids. After an eyelid lift, the eyes are unburdened by excess skin and fat that have distorted their shape, and the result is a more rested, youthful, and alert look. If most of the darkness under the eyes was from shadows, caused from bulges of fat tissue, the shadows will be eliminated; this will further freshen the eyes.

Note that an eyelid lift alone is not intended to correct fine lines or wrinkles around the eyes. However, skin rejuvenation treatments are available to diminish these wrinkles.

Also, an eyelid lift will not correct dark circles under the eyes if the circles are caused by the muscle and other tissues showing through thin skin.

Are You a Candidate for an Eyelid Lift?

Are your upper lids sagging? Are your lower lids puffy? If so, and you are in generally good health, you are likely a candidate for eyelid surgery.

People in a wide range of ages choose to have eyelid lifts. Sometimes even those in their twenties elect to have an eyelid lift because of a genetic disposition toward droopy or baggy lids. More often, though, individuals in their thirties, forties, and older choose to have their appearance refreshed with eyelid lifts.

You may *not* be a good candidate for an eyelid lift if you have glaucoma, a detached retina, or "severe dry eye," which is the inability to produce sufficient tears. If you have a thyroid disorder, such as hypothyroidism or Graves' disease, eyelid surgery is likely not advisable since these conditions can affect your eyes. Also, if you have had eye surgery or any paralysis in the face, you might not be a good candidate for this surgery. As always, share your complete medical history with your surgeon.

Sometimes people have puffy eyes from allergies. If puffy eyes is the only problem you want corrected, and if it is due only to allergies, you aren't a good candidate for an eyelid lift.

Undergoing an Eyelid Lift

On the morning of the surgery, wash your face well and don't apply any makeup. Take good sunglasses to the surgical center with you, as you'll need them for the trip home. Upon your arrival at the surgical center, you will likely be given an oral sedative to help you relax.

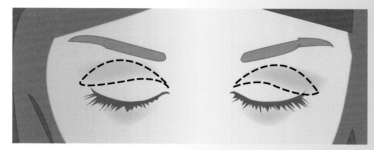

Incision placement for upper eyelid lift

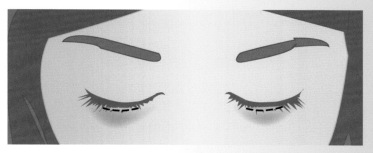

Incision placement, outside the eyelid, for lower eyelid lift

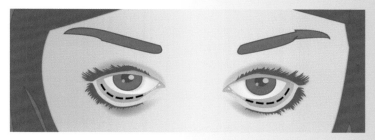

Incision, inside the eyelid, for lower eyelid lift

An eyelid lift procedure is typically an outpatient procedure and takes from thirty minutes to one hour, depending on the experience and skill of the surgeon. If you are having your upper and lower eyelids done together, it's likely that your doctor will lift the upper lids first. If you are having a brow lift with an eyelid lift, your surgeon may perform the brow lift first in order to see how the higher brow position will affect the skin over the eyelids. Eyelid surgery is usually performed under twilight sedation or general anesthesia. The surgeon will also inject a local anesthesia in the eyelid tissues.

Upper Eyelid Lift

For the upper eyelid lift, the surgeon makes incisions in the creases of the upper lids. Through these incisions, the doctor will trim away excess skin and remove extraneous fat and muscle tissue. He or she will also redrape excess skin and muscle. The incisions will be closed with sutures.

Lower Eyelid Lift

To perform a lower eyelid lift, your surgeon will make incisions in the lower lids, about two millimeters below the lashes. These incisions can be transcutaneous, which means through the skin, or transconjunctival, on the inside of the eyelids. The transcutaneous incisions made on the outside of the eyelid result in tiny scars that are barely visible. Skin can be tightened through these same incisions and skin resurfacing can be avoided. A disadvantage, this type of incision can exacerbate dry eyes and alter eye shape.

One advantage of transconjunctival incisions, those being made inside the lower eyelid, is that the tiny scar will be totally hidden. This approach also helps avoid a rare complication called lower eyelid retraction, in which the eyelid becomes lax and in some cases can pull away from the eye. Another advantage of these incisions is that they do not exacerbate dry eyes. However, this approach does not allow for tightening loose skin.

Once the incisions have been made, your surgeon will usually remove the excess fat in the lower lids. This is the fat that has protruded through the soft tissue in the lids, creating bags under the eyes. Sometimes the fat is not removed, but repositioned below the rim of the bone to fill in the area referred to as the tear trough.

Some doctors use a laser or cautery, rather than a scalpel, for lower lid procedures that are performed just to remove fatty deposits. The surgeon will pull down the lower lid and use the laser to make the incision on the inner lid. This means no incision is made on the outer skin; the laser also serves to cauterize the tiny blood vessels, so there is no bleeding.

A laser or electrocautery will be used to remove or sculpt the fat. If skin rejuvenation is being done, the laser can also be used to resurface the skin, diminishing the fine wrinkles around the eyes and removing most skin discoloration. This resurfacing also tightens the skin. When the lower lids are finished, the surgeon will close incisions with sutures.

After Your Eyelid Lift

After the surgery, your doctor will lubricate your eyes with an ointment. You'll spend one to two hours in recovery, during which you will probably feel some tightness and a little tenderness in your eyelids. As you recover, you must have cold compresses applied to reduce swelling. You'll need someone to drive you home, and you'll wear sunglasses to protect you from light and airborne irritants, even if it's cloudy.

Expect your eyes to be sensitive to light and wind for a few days. Specific laser care instructions from your doctor will usually advise keeping your eyelids moist with Vaseline. If your lower lids have been lasered, you'll be advised to wear sunglasses outside for several weeks, not only to protect your eyes from irritants, light, and wind, but also against ultraviolet rays, which can cause the skin to permanently darken. Ask your doctor about sunscreen made especially for eyelids, and use it for a few months.

You'll want to take it easy for the first few days after your procedure. Keep your activities to a minimum for three to five days, and minimize the time you spend reading, watching TV, or sitting at your computer screen. Such activities will cause your eyes to dry out more. Keep your eyes moist by using moistening eyedrops. Most people use them for about a week. For the first week, keep your head elevated with extra pillows; this will help keep the swelling down.

Another way to keep the swelling to a minimum is to use cold compresses around the eyes. Cold cloths or gauze pads soaked in ice water and wrung out work well and can be very soothing.

If you have removable sutures, your surgeon will remove them four to seven days after surgery. Ask your surgeon how soon you can wear eye makeup. Although it takes six to

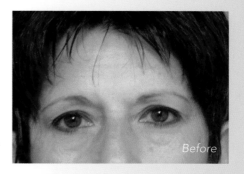

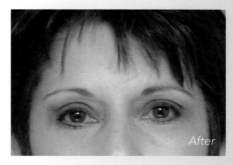

Eyelid lift and brow lift

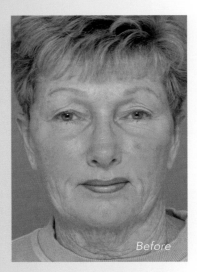

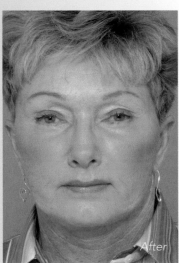

Eyelid lift, brow lift, and facelift

eight months for incisions to heal completely, eyelid incisions heal quickly and are generally inconspicuous after a month.

Avoid strenuous activities and all contact sports for about three weeks. Also avoid lifting and bending, activities that raise your blood pressure.

You won't be able to wear contacts for one to two weeks. Most people return to work and activities in a week to ten days after eyelid surgery.

How Long Will an Eyelid Lift Last?

Generally, an eyelid lift will last approximately ten years. Results will vary among individuals, depending on whether they're smokers, have excess sun explore, or suffer from chronic illness.

Side Effects of an Eyelid Lift

Common side effects from eyelid lifts include temporary swelling around the corners of the eyelids, and minor bruising during the first week. Your eyes might be puffy for a week or two, and you might experience double or blurred vision for a few days. The blurred vision is commonly caused by the ointment used on your incisions. The swelling can temporarily affect your vision as well. Even perfect eyelid incisions may temporarily thicken.

Your eyes might feel dry and gummy for a few weeks to a month or two. This is due to a temporary change in the protective film that covers the eyeball. In the meantime, use eyedrops to moisten your eyes.

You might also develop whiteheads, milia, which are tiny cysts, on the scar line; these may disappear on their own or your doctor may remove them with a fine needle.

Potential Complications of an Eyelid Lift

Any surgery carries with it the possibility of infection and bleeding. With eyelid lifts, there are other potential complications as well, though they are rare:

- Asymmetry in the eyelids
- Trouble fully closing the eyes because too much skin has been lifted. This can be repaired.
- The lower lids may have been pulled down too far. This would require further surgery.

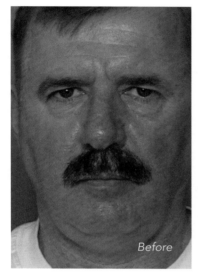

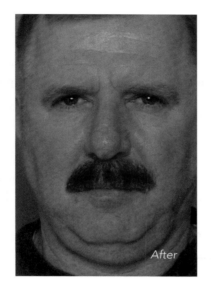

Before · After

Eyelid lift

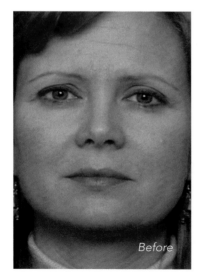

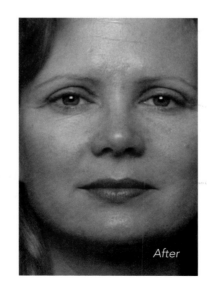

Before · After

Eyelid lift

1. Will lifting my upper lids be enough? Do my lower lids need lifting?

2. For lower lids, do you use a laser?

3. Will my dark circles be removed during a lower eyelift?

4. Where will my incisions be?

5. What will my recovery be like?

6. How soon can I drive?

7. When can I return to work?

8. What are potential complications, and how would they be handled?

9. Will I need other treatments to rejuvenate my eyes?

10. Will the shape of my eyes stay the same?

- Orbital hematoma. The most serious complication of eyelid surgery. It is very obvious because one eye protrudes and is painful.

What Is a Brow Lift?

A brow lift is not about creating high eyebrows. Often only upper eye shape is the goal. A brow lift, also called a forehead lift, is a procedure that elevates the soft tissue and skin of the forehead and brow. The brow lift smoothes lines in the forehead and rejuvenates the brow area, which may have become heavy looking, creating a tired or unhappy look. It is especially effective in rejuvenating the upper eyelids.

Both men and women can benefit from brow lifts. A man typically has a heavier brow than a woman does, but as a woman's brow begins to droop, her brow becomes more masculine. How so? The "shelf" on the outer half of the brow, where the skin drapes the bone, makes the eye feminine and youthful. As the brow droops, this shelf disappears. A brow lift restores youthfulness to the eyes, resulting in a softer, refreshed appearance.

To achieve the look you desire, you may need a brow lift in combination with an eyelid lift. In some cases, either of these procedures alone will not accomplish the rejuvenation you're seeking. Talk to your surgeon about whether you will benefit from one procedure or whether you need both.

Are You a Candidate for a Brow Lift?

You are a good candidate for a brow lift if your brow is low or heavy, contributing to sagging upper eyelids, or if you have lines in your forehead that make you look tired or angry. As mentioned, brow lifts are often combined with eyelid lifts. It is common and often necessary for a cosmetic surgeon to combine a brow lift with a facelift.

Many men assume they can't have a brow lift if they're bald or if they have a receding hairline, but this isn't true. If you are one of these men, talk to your surgeon about the options available for you.

Undergoing a Brow Lift

The *endoscopic brow lift* is the brow lift most commonly performed. It involves fewer and smaller incisions, which are hidden in the hair.

To undergo this procedure, you will likely be given twilight sedation. If you are not having another procedure along with the brow lift, your surgery may take as little as thirty minutes.

To perform an endoscopic brow lift, the surgeon makes from three to five incisions above the hairline; these incisions are one-half inch to an inch long. An endoscope is inserted through one of the incisions and the surgeon views the underlying muscles and tissues on a television monitor that is connected to the endoscope's tiny camera.

Using an instrument inserted through a nearby incision, the doctor lifts the forehead tissues. Once lifted, the tissues are anchored into place by one of several techniques. Some surgeons may anchor the lifted tissues with sutures; others may use tiny titanium screws or small, bioabsorbable plates that dissolve several months later.

When your surgeon has completed the lift, he or she will close the incisions with stitches or small clips. Some surgeons place a bandage, to be worn overnight, around the head.

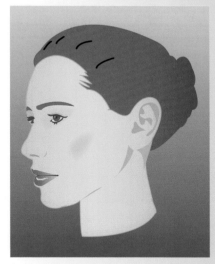

Incision for endoscopic brow lift

How Long Will a Brow Lift Last?

On average, a brow lift should last from five to eight years. Life style factors, including fluctuations in weight, can affect results.

Other Approaches to Brow Lifts

Other brow lift procedures can also be effective in rejuvenating the face by correcting drooping eyebrows and diminishing lines between the eyes and across the forehead.

Coronal Brow Lift

The incisions made for this lift can extend from ear to ear or be primarily limited to the top of the head. During this procedure, one to two centimeters of skin and soft tissue are removed.   Tightening is achieved by suturing a deep strong fibrous layer below the skin called the galea. Then, the scalp skin is closed. This lift offers better control of the brow position and a more long-lasting effect. Muscles between the eyebrows can also be treated. Numbness will be present for about nine months behind the incision on the top of the head.

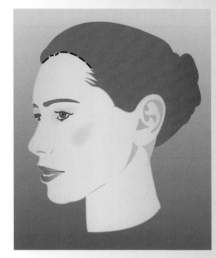

Incision for pretrichial brow lift

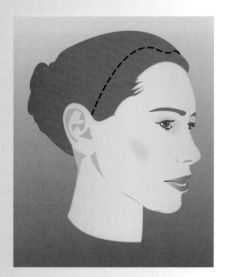

Incision for coronal brow lift

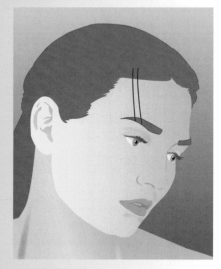

Brow lift with cable threads

Combined Coronal/Endoscopic Brow Lift

Shorter incisions similar to those used with a coronal brow lift are made but are positioned only behind the hairline. Endoscopes and instruments are inserted and similar lifting and between-eyebrow muscle work is done. The lift is then spread across the entire length of the incision instead of being made at only a few points. Since tissue is removed, this lift is longer lasting. Similar to coronal or endoscopic lifts, it will raise the hairline and also produce numbness behind it.

Thread Brow Lift

Contour threads can also be used to lift the brow. To perform a contour thread brow lift, the surgeon makes an incision in the hairline and the skin of the forehead. The skin is lifted. An endoscope may or may not be used with the thread technique. The incision will not be visible after healing because it is hidden in the hairline.

Petrichial Brow Lift

As both men and women age, their hairlines recede. Given this fact, it's important to note that this is the only browlift that lowers, not raises, a forehead hairline. The incision precisely follows the front hairline, weaving in the first few hairs. Great care is taken to bevel or angle the incision, which allows hair to grow through the healing incision line. This incision gives the surgeon the most control over the brow position and heals well. Similarly, muscles can be treated between the eyebrows. As is the case with the coronal brow lift, numbness will be present behind the incision line for about nine months.

Mid-Forehead Brow Lift

For this lift, the surgeon makes an incision in one of the creases in the forehead. This type of lift is intended to lift the eyebrows and not the entire forehead. Tightening is limited since there is no deep anchoring and tension on the skin should be avoided. It may work best for men who have heavy brows and little hair on their heads to conceal scars. It can also be used as a touch-up brow lift. This lift is not commonly used.

Temporal Brow Lift

A *temporal brow lift*, also known as a *lateral brow lift*, lifts the drooping skin of the outer brow line. It does not lift the mid-forehead. To perform this procedure, the surgeon places small, diamond-shaped incisions at the hairline on both sides of the forehead. The

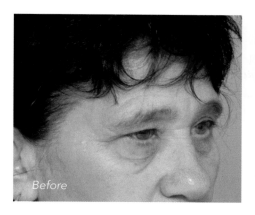
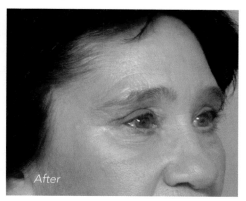

Before

After

Eyelid lift, brow lift, and laser skin resurfacing

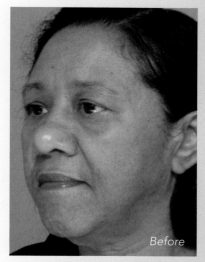

Before

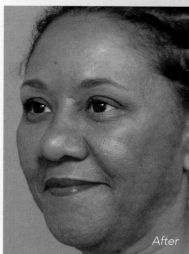

After

Eyelid lift and brow lift

excess skin is removed, lifting the outer corners of the forehead. The scars from a temporal brow lift will be inconspicuous in most people. However, this lift might not hold as long as other lifts.

Direct Brow Lift

In the *direct brow lift,* incisions are made just above the brows. However, even in men with heavy eyebrows, it's difficult to hide the scars, and the incisions can alter the eyebrows to make them look less masculine. There are better options than this older technique.

After a Brow Lift

Once you've returned home, you can use a cold compress to keep the swelling down; when sleeping or resting, use an extra pillow to keep your head elevated.

You'll have a follow-up appointment with your surgeon the next day. During this appointment you will likely have your hair washed by the surgeon's staff, and your surgeon will remove any bandages and check your incisions. Thereafter, you'll be able to shower and shampoo at home. Ask your surgeon how long you should wait before wearing makeup. Some surgeons allow you to wear it the next day; others will suggest that you wait a few days.

Questions to ask your surgeon

1. Will a brow lift alone give me the results I want?

2. What type of brow lift do you recommend?

3. Will I have visible scars?

4. What will my recovery be like?

5. When can I return to work?

6. What will happen to my hairline?

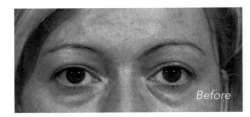
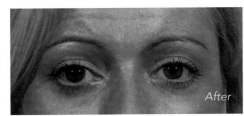

Upper and lower eyelid lift

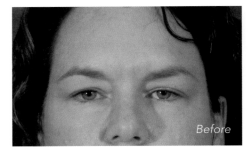
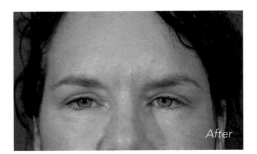

Eyelid lift

You'll have any stitches or staples removed in seven to ten days. If screws were used, these screws will be removed in about two weeks. As mentioned, however, newer procedures use a dissolvable device so that no screw removal is required.

Usually, you can go back to work within a week; however, you should not do any heavy lifting or hard exercise for a few weeks. After that, you can resume your normal exercise. After a brow lift, you can continue to wear contact lenses. If small amounts of hair shed at the incision site, it should grow back within a few weeks or months. Most visible signs of surgery should be gone within about three weeks.

Side Effects of a Brow Lift

With a brow lift, you can expect some minor swelling and bruising around the forehead, cheeks, and eyes. You may experience mild discomfort, for which you can be prescribed pain medication. Also for lifts other than endoscopic, you might experience som scalp itching along the incision; this could last a few weeks to a few months. Any numbness or tingling that you feel after the surgery should subside; in some cases the numbness persists.

Potential Complications of a Brow Lift

Complications that can occur after a brow lift include areas of numbness due to sensory nerve injury. Rarely, nerve injury can also cause loss of movement of the muscles that raise the eyebrows or wrinkle the forehead. It is possible for the procedure to result in asymmetry, with one or both brows appearing too high; however, this usually evens out as healing progresses. Hair loss is possible around incisions.

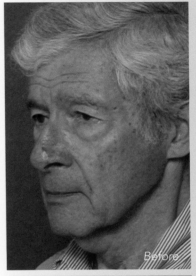

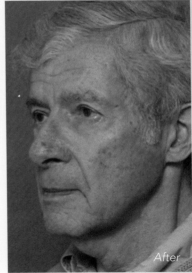

Eyelid lift

CHAPTER ELEVEN

Skin Rejuvenation

11

Skin Rejuvenation

As the years roll by, not only does our skin begin to sag, but the surface of our skin also ages. As mentioned earlier, these changes start by age thirty, when we start to lose that youthful glow. In addition to natural aging, other factors also play a role in how our outer skin looks as we age. These include sun damage, acne, nutrition, and whether or not we've smoked or consumed alcohol.

But today, a variety of treatments are available to rejuvenate your skin. You've probably heard of many of them, such as laser skin resurfacing, chemical peels, Botox injections, microdermabrasion, thermoplasty, and wrinkle fillers. The number of individuals undergoing such nonsurgical procedures has skyrocketed in recent years.

Treating the Skin with Lasers

The use of lasers to treat skin problems is one of the remarkable developments in cosmetic surgery in recent years. How do lasers work? A laser emits a narrow beam of light, which transmits an extreme heat. The heat vaporizes skin imperfections. Since our bodies are 70 percent water, when the laser beam hits skin tissue, the water molecules in the skin cells absorb the beam and their temperature goes to twice that of boiling; this causes the tissue to vaporize without burning the patient. The laser instrument is computer driven, so the surgeon is able to carefully control the intensity of the light, the energy and density of the beam, and the length of time it contacts the skin.

There are two basic types of lasers used in treating the skin. *Ablative lasers* are used in more aggressive treatments, such as laser skin resurfacing. These lasers are capable of ablating, or completely removing, a layer of skin. *Nonablative lasers* are less aggressive and are used to treat skin imperfections without damaging the surface skin.

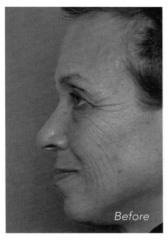
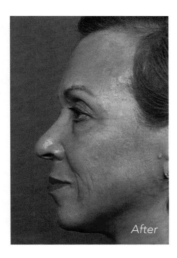

Before

After

Laser skin rejuvenation

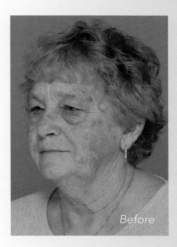

Before

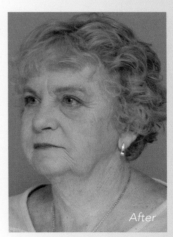

After

Laser skin resurfacing
and eyelid lift

Undergoing Laser Skin Resurfacing

An ablative laser is used to totally resurface the skin, removing sun damage and fine wrinkles. (See the Glogau chart in this chapter for information on sun-damaged skin). This treatment leaves a smoother, brighter, firmer skin. In effect, the laser burns off the damaged skin and allows new skin to take its place. This laser also transmits heat deeper into the skin, causing tightening of the collagen bundles and the formation of new collagen. As a result, the skin smoothes and tightens.

Ablative laser resurfacing takes from thirty to sixty minutes, depending on the amount of resurfacing being done. It is usually performed in a surgical suite. Typically you will receive a nerve block or twilight sedation, in which you are not unconscious but feel no pain. This is given through an IV. Your skin will be cleansed and your heart, blood pressure, and blood oxygen level will be monitored.

Using a CO_2 laser, the surgeon passes the laser beam over your skin. The laser removes the epidermis, the outer skin, and part of the upper dermis below it. After a pass with the

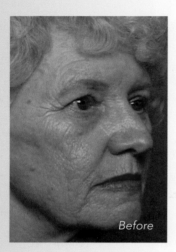

Before

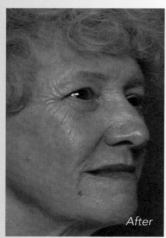

After

Laser skin resurfacing

laser, your face will be wiped to cool the skin and remove the dead tissue. Some areas of the face might take several passes.

LASERS USED IN SKIN REJUVENATION	
ABLATIVE LASERS	
Carbon Dioxide (CO_2)	Rejuvenates sun-damaged skin by resurfacing the top layer. Can also soften wrinkles and diminish crow's-feet and upper lip lines.
Erbium	Resurfaces the top layer of skin and tightens underlying tissue. Stimulates collagen growth, diminishes wrinkles, and improves minor scars and discolorations.
NONABLATIVE LASERS	
Neodymium	Improves skin firmness and elasticity. Also removes dark pigment and unwanted hair.
Yellow Light	Removes port-wine stains, rosacea, and enlarged blood vessels. Treats some raised scars and removes red, orange, and yellow tattoo pigments.
Alexandrite and Ruby	Alexandrite is used to remove hair on people with darker skin. Ruby works best on those with pale skin and dark hair. Both are used in tattoo removal. Alexandrite is used to remove black, blue, and green; Ruby removes black, purple, violet, and other dark colors.
Diode	Removes hair in people with fair skin and dark hair. Also used to treat spider veins and flat brown spots.

Following the procedure, the treated skin will be wrapped in a sterile dressing and you'll spend an hour or two in recovery, after which you'll need a caregiver to drive you home.

In recent years, surgeons have begun spraying platelet gel over the surface of the patient's face after the procedure, to help speed healing. This gel will cause the face to become bright red. Many surgeons also cover the face with a transparent dressing, similar to plastic wrap you use in the kitchen.

Are You a Candidate for Laser Skin Resurfacing?

Laser resurfacing is not recommended for people who have active acne or who have light skin as defined by the Fitzpatrick skin type classification. The laser can cause *hypopigmentation*, or splotches of white, in these people. On the other end of the spectrum, those with dark skin are at risk for *hyperpigmentation*, splotches of dark skin.

FITZPATRICK CLASSIFICATION OF SKIN TYPE

Skin Type	Description	Reaction to Sun
I	Pale white or freckled	Always burns, never tans
II	White	Always burns easily, tans minimally
III	White to light brown	Burns moderately, tans uniformly
IV	Moderate brown	Burns minimally, always tans well
V	Dark brown	Rarely burns, tans profusely
VI	Very dark brown to black	Never burns

After Laser Skin Resurfacing

A few days after the procedure you'll return to the surgeon's office to have any dressings removed. (Not all surgeons apply dressings.) Your skin should be healed within a week; the new layer of skin will be smooth and tight, and is usually a light pink. The skin will be pink for six to eight weeks, depending on the depth of the ablation. New collagen, below the surface of the skin, forms in three to six months, creating a thicker outer skin, which helps reduce wrinkles.

Your doctor will guide you in properly caring for your skin, including the use of ointments, replacing the protective dressing as needed, washing with a special soap that he or she provides, and using generous amounts of sunscreen.

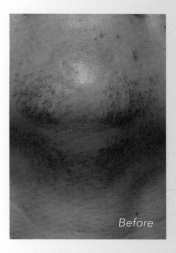

Before

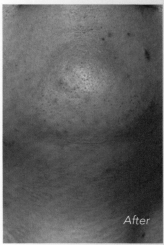

After

Laser hair removal

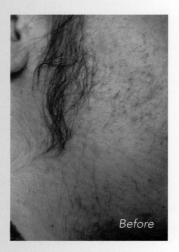

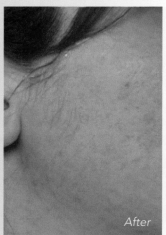

Before

After

Laser hair removal

As you heal, you'll experience some itching; also expect the treated area to be tender and swollen for several days to a week. You can apply makeup seven to ten days after the procedure.

The results of laser skin resurfacing often last anywhere from five to ten years. Wrinkles around the eyes and lips tend to return first, but good skin care can prolong the effects of the resurfacing.

Nonablataive Laser Treatments for Skin

Nonablative lasers, the less aggressive ones, are used to remove spider veins, age spots, warts, and birthmarks; these lasers can also improve facial scars by 10 to 20 percent. Nonablative lasers also firm and tone the skin by stimulating the collagen layer just under the epidermis. As new collagen forms, wrinkles around the eyes, upper lips, cheeks, and forehead are reduced or eliminated.

These lasers are also used to remove dark facial hair, though they are not effective in removing blond, red, or gray hair, because these colors lack the pigment that nonablative lasers affect. Based on your skin condition, your doctor can tell you whether you are better suited for ablative or nonablative resurfacing.

Nonablative treatments are done in your doctor's office, and are often performed by a technician. Your skin will be cleansed and you will wear protective eye goggles. Whether or not you need a topical anesthetic depends on the type of skin problem being treated. For example, removal of an age spot may produce a short stinging sensation, but no anesthetic is required. For other treatments you may receive a topical numbing cream or perhaps an injection of lidocaine.

The treatment takes anywhere from fifteen to forty-five minutes. Afterward, you might be given a cold gel pack to cool your face.

After a Nonablative Laser Treatment

Recovery is very simple after nonablative treatments. There is essentially no swelling, and you can return immediately to normal activities. Although some lasers will leave no discoloration, others may leave a temporary reddish-purple spot, depending on the type of skin imperfection treated and the type of laser used. This spot should fade in seven to fourteen days. In the meantime, you can use makeup, but be sure to ask your doctor about what kinds are appropriate. Avoid picking or scratching the treated areas as they heal.

Potential Complications

With ablative laser treatments, such as skin resurfacing, there is a risk of infection, just as there would be with any such medical procedure. However, antibiotics greatly reduce the likelihood of that occurring. If you should have an undiagnosed case of herpes simplex virus in the skin, a laser treatment could activate the virus and result in scarring.

The risk of complications with nonablative laser treatments is minimal. Still, there is a risk of scarring, especially if the surgeon is not experienced. As mentioned earlier, there is a possibility of developing blotches of white (or dark) on the skin, if patients are not carefully screened for skin type.

GLOGAU CLASSIFICATION OF SUN DAMAGE TO SKIN			
Group	Degree of Sun Damage	Age Range	Appearance
I	Mild	25–35 years old	No keratosis, little scarring or wrinkling. Little or no makeup needed.
II	Moderate	35–50 years old	Early wrinkling, mild scarring and/or discoloration. Little makeup needed.
III	Advanced	50–65 years old	Keratosis, wrinkles, discoloration, telangiectasias (swollen blood vessels). Always wears makeup.
IV	Severe	65–75 years old	Keratosis, deep wrinkles, skin laxity, discoloration, scarring. Makeup is caked.

Uses for Nonablative Lasers

- Firm and tone the skin
- Remove age spots
- Remove spider veins
- Remove port-wine birthmarks
- Reduce redness from rosacea
- Remove unwanted hair
- Reduce acne scars and other minor scars
- Remove warts
- Remove tattoos

What Is a Chemical Peel?

A chemical peel is a procedure in which a chemical solution is applied to the face to remove damaged layers of skin. A peel can improve uneven skin pigmentation and blemishes. It won't tighten skin or slow the aging process, but it will improve the skin's texture and surface. Peels also boost collagen production, which can help prevent new wrinkles from forming. The skin appears fresher and smoother, and age spots and precancerous lesions are eliminated.

Generally, the types of acids used in chemical peels are alpha hydroxy, trichloroacetic, or phenol. Peels can also contain anti-acne agents, melanin inhibitors to prohibit the formation of skin discoloration or brown spots, and hormones to improve skin moisture and plumpness.

Before the Peel

Your doctor will provide you with a cleanser to use for a few weeks before your peel. If you are having a light peel, you will likely be instructed to discontinue any use of Retin-A cream since it could intensify the penetration of the chemical, something not needed for the light peel.

However, if you are having a medium, modified deep, or deep peel, your surgeon may prescribe Retin-A to exfoliate the skin and allow for the solution to penetrate more deeply. Proper skin care prior to the procedure will help the skin peel more evenly and reduce the likelihood of uneven coloring. To aid in the healing process, your doctor will likely recommend that you stop smoking and drinking for at least a week prior to your treatment.

Light Peel

If you want to rejuvenate tired-looking skin, you're a likely candidate for a light chemical peel. A light peel can be done on any skin type. It can improve the appearance of pigment changes, acne scars, mild sun damage, and fine wrinkles. Typically performed in your doctor's office, a light peel uses alpha hydroxy acids, which produce a mild formula. A mild peel might need to be performed several times to achieve the desired effect.

A solvent will be used to cleanse your face, and your doctor might lightly abrade your skin to remove dead cells and aid in the penetration of the chemicals. Once this is done, the chemical solution will be applied with a cotton pad or brush. The solution will be on your face for two to seven minutes. You'll feel a minor stinging, but it usually doesn't require any pain medication. Depending on the chemical used, your face might be rinsed thoroughly after the treatment, after which moisturizing cream will be applied.

Your skin might be somewhat pink and a little dry for a few days. You can wear makeup immediately after your light peel. There's no downtime with this recovery; you can return to work immediately. Rich moisturizers will help soothe your skin.

Medium Peel

If you're fair-skinned, you could be a candidate for a medium peel. These peels aren't recommended for people with dark skin or with oily skin. Medium peels involve the use of trichloroacetic acid, which penetrates deeper than the acid used in light peels. A medium peel can diminish or eliminate mild to moderate wrinkles, long-term sun damage, pigment changes, and precancerous skin lesions.

This procedure is performed in your doctor's office; you may be given a mild sedative or pain medication prior to the peel. The peel itself is similar to a light peel, but the chemical is left on your face longer, for a total of about ten to fifteen minutes. As the chemical solution removes dead skin cells, your skin temporarily turns frosty white. In some medical practices, a fan is aimed at your face to soothe the burning sensation you will feel during this peel.

After a Medium Peel

Once the peel is finished, you will have little or no pain, but it takes up to two weeks before you feel presentable. Until then, your face will be red and the skin will peel. You might experience some soft, crusty areas during the first several days, especially in areas that received the greatest penetration. To aid in the healing, make sure you don't pick at the crust. With makeup, you might feel okay to go out after a week or so.

You'll cleanse with products your doctor gives you, applying ointments to soothe the skin and aid the healing. When you go outdoors, you will need a good sunblock to protect your skin.

Modified Deep Peel

Today, the traditional deep peels, which use the chemical phenol, are not performed as much as they once were. These peels were painful and required a lengthy recuperation

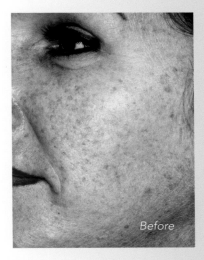

Before

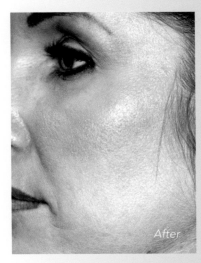

After

Modified deep chemical peel

time. A newer peel—the modified deep peel—is now used by many cosmetic surgeons, using less-caustic products such as liquid soap, crotin oil, phenol, and water. Since a greater amount of crotin oil is used and less phenol, these peels are safer than traditional deep peels, and have a much quicker recovery time. The modified deep peel achieves good results without the severe side effects of a deep peel.

A modified deep peel can treat severe wrinkles, long-term sun damage, pronounced pigment changes, and skin lesions and growths. It is a more aggressive procedure than light and medium peels, and it is performed with the patient receiving twilight anesthesia in a surgical facility.

Once your skin is cleansed, the solution is applied to your face, with heavier applications applied around the eyes and mouth, where fine lines are usually more concentrated. The procedure takes between fifteen and thirty minutes, after which your face will be covered with an emollient cream or petroleum jelly. As you come to, you will feel like you have a severe sunburn. You will be given pain medication, recover for an hour or two, and then you can be driven home.

After a Modified Deep Peel

Since the modified deep peel procedure goes deeper, the recovery takes longer. Your face will be swollen for a day or two. You might not feel like talking for the first few days, because you will be uncomfortable when you move your face. You might experience crusting for about a week. Don't pick at the crusts.

After the first week, you will begin to peel as you would after a severe sunburn. Your doctor will give you ointments to apply; keeping your face moist will lessen the pain and aid in the healing. You can also be prescribed pain medication.

You can wear makeup after the first week or so to camouflage the redness. After about a month, your new skin will feel rough or even finely wrinkled. Over the next six to eight weeks, this roughness will smooth out. As your new skin appears, it might be slightly lighter than before.

As you're recovering from a modified deep or deep peel, you will gently cleanse your face with your fingertips and cool water, patting your face dry with a clean towel. To help keep the swelling down, when sleeping use several pillows to elevate your head for the first several nights.

You should ease back into exercise after six to eight weeks, and avoid outdoor activities for at least two months.

How Long Will a Peel Last?

A light peel is usually done in a series of six to twelve treatments over a month's time. Some patients return every two or three months for a maintenance treatment. To maintain the benefits, a light peel should be repeated at least once a year.

A medium peel might be repeated in three to five years. A modified deep or deep peel will last for many years and generally is not repeated.

Side Effects and Potential Complications

With a light peel, you might get some lingering dryness of skin. The deeper the peel, the greater this risk. Skin redness can be severe, depending on the depth of the peel and the skin type; this redness can last several months.

In addition, a peel, especially a deeper one, can result in the color of the skin changing, and there is a risk of the treated areas being noticeable because of this color change. Also, if you have a history of herpes, you are more prone to infection than others, and a peel could trigger a new outbreak. You might also become more sensitive to the sun after a peel. Make sure you wear a strong sunblock hereafter.

With the deeper peels that use phenol, there is a risk of heart rhythm disturbances and kidney damage. This risk is reduced by careful monitoring of the amount of phenol used, as well as monitoring the heart during the procedure.

Deep peels are not recommended for people who are a skin type IV, V, or VI on the Fitzpatrick Classification scale. If you fall into one of these categories, ask your doctor about alternative procedures.

Other Skin Rejuvenation Procedures

Microdermabrasion

Microdermabrasion is a procedure that uses fine granules or crystals to remove dead skin cells from the surface of the skin. These crystals or granules are sprayed from a small wand. The crystals exfoliate the top layer of skin and then vacuum the dead skin cells. Think

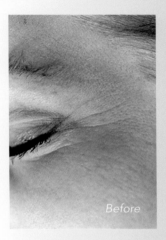
Before

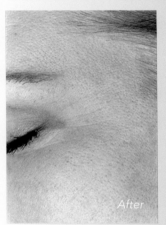
After

Courtesy of Genesis Biosystems

After six weekly treatments, microdermabrasion has stimulated underlying collagen, resulting in softening of fine lines.

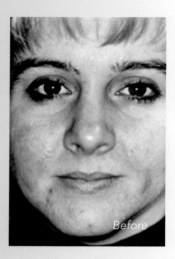
Before

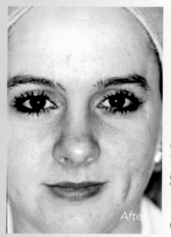
After

Courtesy of Genesis Biosystems

After eight weekly microdermabrasion treatments for active acne

of it as a "mini-sandblasting" of your face. The procedure is painless—some describe it as feeling like light sandpaper being gently rubbed against the skin. For maximum results, you'll need several treatments, one per week, over several weeks.

As microdermabrasion removes the topmost layer of skin, which is mostly composed of dead skin cells, it also removes pore-clogging debris. The result is a fresher, smoother skin and a more even skin tone. The treatment will also repair minor sun damage, soften fine lines, and reduce age spots and blemishes. Because it is effective in cleaning the pores, microdermabrasion is effective in treating acne. It also softens shallow acne scars, but will not eliminate deep scarring.

A treatment can be performed over a lunch hour; it takes twenty to thirty minutes and doesn't require any anesthesia. You can return to work or other activities immediately. Your face, which will feel slightly sunburned or wind burned for a few hours after a treatment, will fully recover within twenty-four hours. You should apply moisturizers to your face. Ask your doctor what type of makeup you can wear within the first twenty-four hours. After that, you can wear the makeup of your choice. You should avoid the sun for the first week, and be sure to use sunscreen when you are outside.

A microdermabrasion can be used on all skin types with no risk of changing the color of the skin. However, if you have active sores or have recently had a herpes outbreak, you should delay a microdermabrasion treatment; any such treatment may activate the virus.

Botox

Botox Cosmetica, more commonly known as Botox, is one of the most popular cosmetic procedures being performed today. Botox reduces facial wrinkles that form as a result of facial expressions. The Botox blocks signals from the nerves to the muscles, resulting in the muscles not being able to contract. Used in small, diluted amounts, doctors can inject the toxin into specific muscles, causing them to weaken and relax. As a result, the wrinkles that are caused by muscle contraction diminish.

The only official, FDA-approved use of Botox is for "frown lines" in the glabella region—the area between the eyebrows. However, it is also used to soften wrinkles in the forehead, around the eyes, and in the neck area, and vertical lines above the lip. Botox has no effect on wrinkles caused by sun damage and gravity.

The treatment takes only minutes and requires no anesthesia. Your doctor will use a fine needle to inject multiple areas. You may be given an ice pack after the treatment to diminish the minor discomfort. You will see the results of a Botox treatment within one to two days; however, it may take up to ten days before you see the full effect.

Botox treatments usually last for three to six months. The lines will gradually begin to reappear, though after several treatments they might return with less severity than before.

Side effects include temporary minor bruising and, in rare cases, headaches for a day or two. Another rare effect is eyelid drooping, which usually lasts no more than three weeks. If you are pregnant, breast-feeding, or have a neurological disease, you shouldn't use Botox. Also, Botox may not be recommended for older patients.

Thermoplasty

Thermoplasty, more commonly known as *thermage*, is a procedure that tightens and lifts the skin. It uses radio frequency to apply intense heat to underlying skin while outer skin layers are cooled with cryogen spray. This action tightens the underlying collagen network, which causes your skin to tighten and lift. The process also stimulates the formation of new collagen, which helps to reduce wrinkles and tighten pores.

You'll likely be given a sedative just prior to the procedure, so you will need to have someone drive you home. You will have virtually no downtime, though you might have some slight swelling for four or five days, and you might feel like you have a sunburn. Temporary bruising and numbness are rare.

Generally, a series of treatments is required, with later touch-ups as needed. The effects can last for several years. This procedure is not recommended for older patients with significant signs of aging.

IPL Photo Rejuvenation

Intense pulsed light (IPL) photo rejuvenation is a noninvasive technique that evens skin tone and texture. It can minimize fine lines and result in smoother, fresher-looking skin. It diminishes brown and red spots, blemishes, rosacea, spider

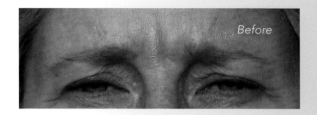

Before

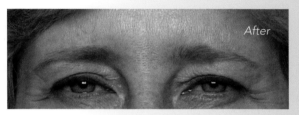

After

Botox injections between the eybrows diminish frown lines.

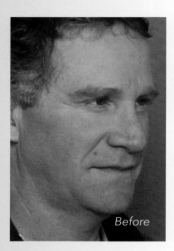

Before

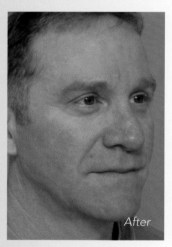

After

Thermage has tightened the underlying collagen, causing the eyebrows to lift.

veins, age spots, sun damage, freckles, enlarged pores, and birthmarks; it can also be used to improve hyperpigmentation (dark splotches).

IPL photo rejuvenation delivers ultraviolet and other types of light in pulses, destroying brown and red spots and darker cells, causing them to fade away. In addition, IPL stimulates collagen production, resulting in firmer, smoother skin.

It is especially important for you to stay out of the sun for several weeks before and after an IPL treatment since tanning can cause your skin to absorb too much light during the treatment; sun exposure afterward can damage your fresh, new layer of skin.

During the treatment, which lasts from fifteen to forty-five minutes, you'll be asked to wear protective goggles. The surgeon will apply a cold gel and may use a topical anesthetic, though there is only minor discomfort without an anesthetic. The doctor or a technician will deliver the pulsed light through a handheld device.

Typically, a patient will have a series of five or six treatments, about three weeks apart. The treatments are long-lasting, though some people decide to have an annual treatment or two in addition to the initial series.

You might have some slight redness and minor swelling following the treatment; this should last no more than a day or two. Bruising and blistering are rare. Many people return to work immediately following an IPL treatment.

What Are Soft Tissue Fillers?

Today, soft tissue fillers, also known as wrinkle fillers, are popular cosmetic procedures. Soft tissue fillers will plump up wrinkles and creases, blending them into the rest of your skin. Such fillers are commonly used to soften nasolabial folds, forehead lines, crow's-feet, smile lines, frown lines, and wrinkles around the lips. Most of these fillers are delivered by injection; there is a variety of filler materials available to surgeons. Most of the injectable fillers are temporary, and the treatments must be repeated to maintain the effects.

Restylane

Of the soft tissue fillers, Restylane is perhaps the one most commonly used today. Manufactured in a laboratory, this synthetic material contains hyaluronic acid, which is found naturally in our skin. It is part of the skin structure that creates volume and shape to our skin by retaining moisture. As we age, we lose some of this structure.

Restylane diminishes wrinkles by restoring volume. Its molecules draw in water, causing the underlying tissues to swell, resulting in fewer wrinkles on the skin's surface. As the body reabsorbs the additional hyaluronic acids, the effects begin to fade, and the procedure will need to be repeated. A treatment generally lasts from six to twelve months.

Surgeons inject Restylane just under the skin, generally without anesthetics. You might experience mild itching, redness, pain, and swelling, but, generally, people return immediately to work or to other activities. Because hyaluronic acid is found naturally in our cells, there is little risk of allergic reaction.

Hylaform

Another injectable filler, Hylaform is a sticky, adhesive, elastic gel, which also contains hyaluronic acid. It is similar to Restylane. However, it is not a synthetic material—it's made from animal products—but it does not require a pretest for allergic reactions.

Depending on the depth of the wrinkles, an initial treatment might be followed by a second treatment about a month later. Most treatments last from six to eight months.

The results with Hylaform are instantaneous, and while mild redness, itching, pain, and swelling might occur, most people return immediately to work.

Radiesse

Radiesse is a longer-lasting injectable filler. It is a synthetic form of calcium hydroxylapatite, a mineral found in our bones and teeth. The particles in the material form a scaffold through which your body's own collagen grows, causing the tissues to plump up, resulting in a smoother skin surface. Its effects can last for several months to a year, although it has been known to last longer in some patients.

Radiesse is injected after your doctor uses a numbing cream or local anesthetic. Because it contains a mineral that occurs naturally in our bodies, it causes no allergic reactions.

Sculptra

Sculptra is an injectable filler used to restore volume rather than reduce wrinkles. It fills in areas below the skin where natural fat has been lost. Sculptra adds volume to

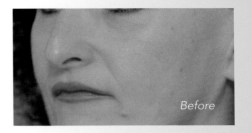
Before

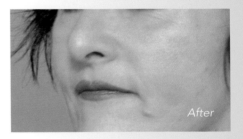
After

Soft tissue filler in nasolabial folds

Glossary

ablative: refers to a type of skin resurfacing in which lasers are used. Ablative treatments resurface the top layer of skin.

blepharoplasty: a procedure also known as an eyelid lift. It provides a more rested, youthful, alert look by removing excess skin, muscle, and fat from around the eyes. The procedure can also help you see better if you have excess skin drooping around the corners of your eyes.

collagen: a fibrous protein that holds the components of the dermis in place.

composite facelift: a variation of a deep-plane facelift. Like the deep-plane, it lifts and repositions skin, fat, and muscle, and it includes lifting the muscles around the lower eyelids as well.

coronal brow lift: uses an incision that goes from ear to ear across the top of the head.

deep-plane facelift: is done at a level (plane) of the face where the majority of aging is occurring. It allows the thick, strong, fibrous tissue layer to be repositioned and tightened, rather than the skin to be pulled, to achieve the desired cosmetic outcome.

dermis: the layer of skin under the epidermis. It contains blood vessels, lymph vessels, hair follicles, and sweat glands. It also contains collagen and elastin, proteins that give your skin its strength and elasticity.

direct brow lift: a brow lift that is sometimes used for men with heavy eyebrows. Incisions are made in the eyebrows, but scarring often shows and the eyebrows are altered.

elastin: a rubbery protein in the skin that helps to return the dermis to normal after an injury.

endoscope: a tiny fiber-optic lens that is inserted through easily hidden incisions in the mouth and temple. The lens is attached to a camera; the physician can view a monitor in the operating room to see inside the skin, and is able to operate by manipulating the endoscope's tools externally.

endoscopic brow lift: the brow lift preferred by most doctors. Three to five small incisions are placed above the hairline. An endoscope is inserted through one of the incisions and the doctor views the muscles and tissues on a monitor that is connected to the endoscope's tiny camera.

epidermis: the outer layer of skin. It actually consists of several layers. As the cells move up through these layers, they form the outer surface of our skin, which is the toughest part.

erbium: an erbium laser is used for ablative skin resurfacing.

hematoma: occurs when blood pools and clots within the tissue under the skin.

hyaluronic acid: a component of connective tissue whose function is to cushion and lubricate. Also called hyaluronan.

hypopigmentation: less color than normal in the skin's pigment. This can be an issue in laser resurfacing for people with dark skin—meaning there will be less pigment, or color, in the areas resurfaced.

intense pulsed light (IPL) photo rejuvenation: a noninvasive technique in which ultraviolet and other types of light are delivered in pulses, destroying brown and red spots and darker cells, causing them to fade away. It can minimize fine lines and result in smoother, fresher-looking skin. It is useful on brown and red spots, blemishes, rosacea, spider veins, age spots, sun damage, freckles, enlarged pores, and birthmarks, and can also be used to improve hyperpigmentation.

mentoplasty: a procedure to augment a receding chin.

microdermabrasion: a procedure in which fine granules or crystals are used to remove dead skin cells on the top layer of skin.

midface lift: a procedure that is carried out to restore a more youthful appearance to the midface area by raising and repositioning the soft tissues between the eyes and the mouth. A midface lift is especially effective in correcting the fold around the nose, known as the nasal furrow.

mid-forehead brow lift: a brow lift sometimes used for bald men. This lift uses an incision that is placed in a deep furrow in the forehead.

mini facelift: a lift that is generally performed on people in their mid-forties or younger. It removes less skin than standard facelifts.

nasolabial fold: the groove that extends from the corner of the nose, around the mouth, and down around the chin.

necrosis: death of skin tissue. Necrosis is more likely to happen in a smoker.

nonablative: refers to a type of skin resurfacing in which lasers are used. Nonablative lasers leave the top layer unharmed.

petrichial brow lift: a brow lift used for people with high foreheads. This incision is made a the edge of the hairline.

photoaging: premature wrinkling due to excessive sun exposure.

platysma muscle: a thin muscle that extends from jawbone to collarbone.

retrognathia: a deficiency in the amount of projection in the chin.

rhytidectomy: facelift.

seroma: a collection of clear fluid under the skin. Can be prevented by placing drainage tubes at the time of the surgery, or by draining with a needle in a postoperative visit.

SMAS: subcutaneous musculoaponeurotic system.

SMAS facelift: sometimes referred to as a two-layer facelift. Surgeons lift two layers: the skin and the SMAS, the thin layer of muscles underneath the skin.

standard facelift: a facelift in which the surgeon repositions the cheeks and neck.

subcutaneous region: layer of skin underneath the dermis. It is made up of collagen and fat cells. This layer insulates our bodies, holding in the heat and acting as a shock absorber for the muscle and bone underneath. It also fills out the skin, giving it its plumpness.

subperiosteal facelift: see deep-plane facelift.

temporal brow lift: uses small, diamond-shaped incisions placed at the hairline on either side of the forehead.

thermoplasty: a procedure that uses radio frequency to apply intense heat to underlying skin while outer skin layers are cooled with cryogen spray. This tightens the collagen network, which causes the skin to tighten and lift.

thread facelift: a minimally invasive lift that uses barbed sutures under the skin to pull and lift it.

transconjunctival: an incision made on the inside of the eyelids.

transcutaneous: an incision through the skin.

trichophytic brow lift: uses an incision a few millimeters inside the hairline. The incision is placed in a beveled manner, through which the hair will regrow.

Resources

American Academy of Facial Plastic and Reconstructive Surgery

310 South Henry Street
Alexandria, VA 22314
Phone: 703-299-9291 or 800-332-FACE
Fax: 703-299-8898
www.facial-plastic-surgery.org

Founded in 1964, the American Academy of Facial Plastic and Reconstructive Surgery (AAFPRS) represents more than 2,700 facial plastic and reconstructive surgeons throughout the world. Among the objectives listed in their mission statement: To promote the highest quality facial plastic surgery through education, dissemination of professional information, and the establishment of professional standards. The AAFPRS is a National Medical Specialty Society of the American Medical Association. AAFPRS members are board-certified surgeons whose focus is surgery of the face, head, and neck. The Web site offers a "virtual exam"—an interactive feature that highlights the most common areas in which facial cosmetic procedures are performed. The online Patient Information Series explains procedures, helps you determine whether they're right for you, and lets you know what to expect. Also on the site are FAQs, before-and-after photos, a physician finder, and a quarterly online magazine.

American Board of Facial Plastic and Reconstructive Surgery

115C South St. Asaph Street
Alexandria, VA 22314
Phone: 703-549-3223
Fax: 703-549-3357
E-mail: tshill@abfprs.org
www.abfprs.org

This organization's mission is to improve the quality of facial plastic surgery available to the public by measuring the qualifications of candidate surgeons against certain rigorous standards. To be considered for membership, a physician must complete a residency program, be in practice a minimum of two years, have 100 operative reports accepted by a peer-review committee, successfully pass an eight-hour written and oral examination, hold the appropriate licensure, and adhere to the ABFPRS Code of Ethics.

American Board of Medical Specialties

1007 Church Street
Suite 404
Evanston, IL 60201-5913
Phone: 847-491-9091
Fax: 847-328-3596
www.abms.org

The American Board of Medical Specialties (ABMS) is an organization of twenty-four approved medical specialty boards. The intent of the certification of physicians is to provide assurance to the public that those certified by an ABMS member board have successfully completed an approved training program and an evaluation process assessing their ability to provide quality patient care in their specialty. Their

Web site explains how specialists are trained and certified; it also offers a search feature for finding certified physicians.

American Board of Otolaryngology

5615 Kirby Drive
Suite 600
Houston, TX 77005
Phone: 713-850-0399
Fax: 713-850-1104
www.aboto.org

Founded in 1924, the American Board of Otolaryngology maintains high standards in the field with the education and examination of ear, nose, and throat physicians. The organization offers subspecialty certificates, including a certificate in plastic surgery of the head and neck. The board's Web site verifies physician certification but doesn't offer referrals. The organization also publishes patient education brochures made available in the offices of its diplomates.

American Board of Plastic Surgery

Seven Penn Center
1635 Market Street
Suite 400
Philadelphia, PA 19103-2204
Phone: 215-587-9322
Fax: 215-587-9622
www.abplsurg.org

The mission of the American Board of Plastic Surgery is to promote safe, ethical, efficacious plastic surgery to the public by maintaining high standards for the education, examination, and certification of plastic surgeons as specialists and subspecialists. Primarily for physicians, the board's Web site includes FAQs explaining how doctors become board-certified and describing differences among licensure, certification, and accreditation.

American Society for Aesthetic Plastic Surgery

11081 Winners Circle
Los Alamitos, CA 90720
Phone: 888-ASAPS-11 (physician referrals)
www.surgery.org

Founded in 1967, ASAPS is a professional organization of plastic surgeons, certified by the American Board of Plastic Surgery, who specialize in cosmetic plastic surgery. The organization has more than two thousand members in the United States and Canada, as well as corresponding members in many other countries. The Web site offers an "Ask an ASAPS Surgeon" feature, as well as news, updates, and consumer-oriented reports on surgical and nonsurgical procedures. The site also has a "Find-a-Surgeon" feature. You'll also find numerous articles and procedure descriptions, some in both English and Spanish.

American Society of Plastic Surgeons

444 East Algonquin Road
Arlington Heights, IL 60005
Phone: 847-228-9900, 888-4-PLASTIC, or 888-475-2784 (physician referrals)
www.plasticsurgery.org

The American Society of Plastic Surgeons (ASPS) is the largest plastic surgery specialty organization in the world. Founded in 1931, the society is composed of board-certified plastic surgeons who perform cosmetic and reconstructive surgery. The mission of the ASPS is to advance quality care to plastic surgery patients by encouraging high standards of training, ethics, physician practice, and research in plastic surgery. The society advocates for patient safety, such as encouraging its members to operate in surgical facilities that have passed rigorous external review of equipment and staffing. The society works in concert with the Plastic Surgery Educational Foundation, founded in 1948, which supports research and educational programs for plastic surgeons. On the society's Web site are FAQs, a history of plastic surgery, a surgeon finder, capsule descriptions of procedures, patient profiles, a photo gallery, and cost information.

**Canadian Academy of Facial Plastic
& Reconstructive Surgery**

600 University Avenue
Suite 401
Mount Sinai Hospital
Toronto, Ontario M5G 1X5
Canada
Phone: 905-569-6965 or 800-545-8864
Fax: 905-569-6960
www.facialcosmeticsurgery.org

The Canadian Academy of Facial Plastic and Reconstructive Surgery (CAFPRS) is an international nonprofit medical society incorporated under the federal laws of Canada. Members of CAFPRS are specialists certified by the Royal College of Physicians and Surgeons of Canada or its equivalent and have met high standards of training and experience in cosmetic and plastic surgery of the face and neck.

U.S. National Library of Medicine

8600 Rockville Pike
Bethesda, MD 20894
www.nlm.nih.gov
www.nlm.nih.gov/medlineplus (MedlinePlus)

The U.S. National Library of Medicine Web site indexes articles (primarily for scientists and health professionals) from more than 3,500 medical journals. MedlinePlus is consumer oriented and includes information on more than 650 topics (conditions, diseases, and wellness), drug information, a medical encyclopedia and dictionary, news, provider directories, and other resources.

Index

About the Authors

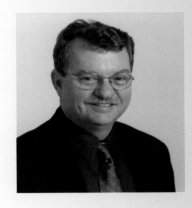

William Truswell, M.D., is a facial plastic surgeon in private practice in Northampton, Massachusetts. He is medical director of the Aesthetic Laser and Cosmetic Surgery Center, which he founded in 1976. He is also coauthor of *Your Complete Guide to Nose Reshaping* (Addicus Books, 2007), *Your Complete Guide to Facial Cosmetic Surgery* (Addicus Books, 2004), and *The Non-Surgical Facelift Book—A Guide to Facial Rejuvenation* (Addicus Books, 2003).

Dr. Truswell received a bachelor of science degree from Hobart College, Geneva, New York. He graduated from the University of Medicine and Dentistry of New Jersey and completed a residency in otolaryngology and facial plastic and reconstructive surgery at the University of Connecticut School of Medicine.

Dr. Truswell is board-certified by the American Board of Facial Plastic and Reconstructive Surgery and the American Board of Otolaryngology. He is a fellow of the American College of Surgeons, the American Academy of Facial Plastic and Reconstructive Surgery, the American Academy of Cosmetic Surgery, the American Academy of Otolaryngology—Head and Neck Surgery, the American Society for Head and Neck Surgery, and the American Academy of Laser Medicine Surgery. He currently serves on the board of directors for the American Academy of Facial Plastic and Reconstructive Surgery and the American Board of Facial Plastic and Reconstructive Surgery.

Dr. Truswell is a clinical instructor in facial plastic surgery in the Division of Otolaryngology, Department of Surgery, University of Connecticut School of Medicine. He is the designer of the Truswell Insertion Instrument for soft tissue implants, manufactured by Marina Medical Corporation.

Dr. Truswell writes articles on facial plastic and reconstructive surgery in medical specialty journals, consults with other professionals for books on facial plastic surgery, and lectures at facial plastic surgery meetings throughout the United States, Europe, and Asia. He has presented papers at the Royal College of Surgeons in London, was a guest lecturer at an annual meeting of the Canadian Academy of Facial Plastic and Reconstructive Surgery, and was on the faculty of the Second World Congress on Advanced Cosmetic Surgery in Ho Chi Minh City, Vietnam, where he was named an Honorary Professor of the Southeast Asia College of Cosmetic Surgery.

To reach Dr. Truswell or to learn more about him and the cosmetic procedures he performs, visit his Web site: **www.truswellplasticsurg.com.**

"That which is truly beautiful is not on the surface. True beauty comes from within and radiates outward. If that is lacking, all that we can create with all our skills as facial plastic surgeons is that which is merely pretty."

—William Truswell, M.D.

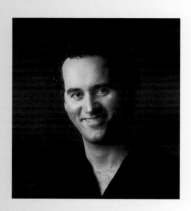

"Facial plastic surgery can offer a tremendous boost to one's self-esteem. With the advances made over the past few years, the entire face can be rejuvenated safely and effectively in less time and often with only local anesthesia. Realistic expectations are a must for anyone considering facial plastic surgery."

—Jon Mendelsohn, M.D.

Jon Mendelsohn, M.D., is a facial plastic surgeon in private practice in Cincinnati, Ohio. He is medical director of the Advanced Cosmetic Surgery & Laser Center. He is also coauthor of *Your Complete Guide to Nose Reshaping* (Addicus Books, 2007), *Your Complete Guide to Facial Cosmetic Surgery* (Addicus Books, 2004), and *The Non-Surgical Facelift Book—A Guide to Facial Rejuvenation* (Addicus Books, 2003).

Dr. Mendelsohn received a bachelor of science degree in molecular biology from Syracuse University. He attended medical school at the State University of New York Health Science Center, Syracuse, and completed a residency there in otolaryngology, head and neck surgery.

Dr. Mendelsohn is board-certified by the American Board of Facial Plastic and Reconstructive Surgery and the American Board of Otolaryngology—Head and Neck Surgery. He is a fellow of the American Academy of Facial Plastic and Reconstructive Surgery, the American College of Surgeons, and the American Academy of Otolaryngology—Head and Neck Surgery.

Dr. Mendelsohn is a member of American Academy of Facial Plastic and Reconstructive Surgery's committees on multimedia and new technologies and devices. He is a national trainer in the use of Botox and Restylane and a regional trainer in the use of autologous platelet gels. He has presented at national conferences on facial plastic surgery and has authored numerous papers and publications on the subject.

To reach Dr. Mendelsohn or to learn more about him and the cosmetic procedures he performs, visit his Web site: **www.351face.com.**

Neil A. Gordon, M.D., F.A.C.S., is a facial plastic surgeon in private practice with offices in Greenwich and Wilton, Connecticut. He is one of a small group of facial plastic surgeons who specialize in the facelift technique called the "deep-plane facelift."

After graduating with highest honors from Albert Einstein College of Medicine in New York, Dr. Gordon completed his internship in general surgery and residency in head and neck surgery at Yale University School of Medicine. He later earned the prestigious fellowship in facial plastic and reconstructive surgery at Tulane University School of Medicine under the instruction of the world renowned facial plastic surgeon, Calvin M. Johnson, M.D.

Dr. Gordon holds double board certification by both the American Board of Facial Plastic and Reconstructive Surgery and the American Board of Otolaryngology. Dr. Gordon sits on the clinical faculty as residency coordinator for facial plastic and reconstructive surgery in the Department of Surgery at Yale University School of Medicine. He is also a current fellow/member of the American Academy of Facial Plastic and Reconstructive Surgery, the American Academy of Otolaryngology—Head and Neck Surgery, Yale Surgical Society, and the American Medical Association. Currently, Dr. Gordon is chairman of the Committee on Patient Safety and Accreditation for the American Academy of Facial Plastic and Reconstructive Surgery.

Dr. Gordon is the director of medical services for the New England Surgical Center, a state-of-the-art facility, which he founded. In addition, he conceived and developed The Retreat at Split Rock, the only specialized surgical facility, spa, inn, and medical offices devoted to cosmetic surgery in the East. He is also a member of both the Connecticut State Medical Society and the Fairfield County Medical Society. Dr. Gordon has written extensively on current concepts in facial plastic surgery and is recognized for his expertise in the most sophisticated techniques in face lifting, brow lifting, and nose surgery. He has often appeared on television and in the print media discussing facial plastic surgery.

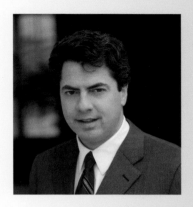

"I believe the best facial plastic surgery procedures are those that go unnoticed by those around you. You shouldn't be able to tell that someone has had cosmetic surgery. My goal as a surgeon is to reverse a patient's signs of aging, without changing the person."

— Neil A. Gordon, M.D.

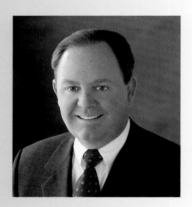

"My goal with facial cosmetic procedures, whether major or minor, is to improve appearance in a measurable way with a natural-looking end result. This should serve to enhance a patient's self-image and their quality of life."

— Harrison C. Putman III, M.D.

Harrison C. "Chris" Putman III, M.D., is a facial plastic surgeon and medical director of the Facial Plastic and Laser Surgery Center in Peoria, Illinois. He also serves on the Medical Executive Committee of the Peoria Day Surgery Center, a multi-specialty surgery center and associated recovery care center for overnight stays. He is an active staff member at OSF Saint Francis Medical Center and at Methodist Medical Center, also in Peoria, Illinois. Dr. Putman received a bachelor of science degree from the University of Notre Dame and his medical degree from Tulane University in New Orleans, Louisiana. His residency training in otolaryngology, facial plastic surgery, and head and neck surgery was also from Tulane University. He is certified by the American Board of Facial Plastic and Reconstructive Surgery and the American Board of Otolaryngology. He is a fellow of the American College of Surgeons, the American Academy of Facial Plastic and Reconstructive Surgery, and the American Society for Laser Medicine and Surgery. He is a past fellow of the American Head and Neck Society. Dr. Putman serves as an assistant clinical professor in the Department of Surgery section of Otolaryngology and Head and Neck Surgery at the University of Illinois College of Medicine in Peoria, Illinois. He is also an associate clinical professor in the Department of Otolaryngology—Head and Neck Surgery at Southern Illinois University Medical School in Springfield, Illinois. He serves as an instructor in facial plastic and reconstructive surgery for this program.

Dr. Putman serves on the board of directors of the American Board of Facial Plastic and Reconstructive Surgery, for which he is credentials committee chairman for the twelve-state Midwest region. He is an oral examiner for the annual certifying examination of the board and also serves on its written exam committee. Dr. Putman is actively involved in teaching facial plastic and reconstructive surgery and laser surgery, as well as lecturing at facial plastic surgery meetings. He serves on the board of directors of several civic and national organizations, including the St. Jude Midwest Affiliate in Peoria, Illinois.

An avid sportsman, Dr. Putman enjoys golf, bird hunting, fresh and saltwater fishing, and other outdoor activities. He and his wife, Mary, enjoy travel, scuba diving, and other activities with their two children, Michelle and Christopher.

Dr. Putman is also coauthor of *Your Complete Guide to Nose Reshaping* (Addicus Books, 2007).

For more information about the procedures performed by Dr. Putman, visit his Web site: **www.putmanfps.com.**

David A. F. Ellis, M.D., is a facial plastic surgeon in private practice at the Art of Facial Surgery, Toronto, Canada. He received his medical degree from the University of Toronto and later became a fellow of the Royal College of Physicians and Surgeons in Otolaryngology (FRSCS). In 1984 Dr. Ellis became a fellow of the American College of Surgery, and in 1989 he received his American board certification in facial plastic and reconstructive surgery.

Dr. Ellis holds the academic rank of professor at the Department of Otolaryngology, University of Toronto, Ontario, Canada. He is a "fellowship mentor" for young surgeons who wish to improve their skills in facial cosmetic surgery, and is also the core lecture coordinator for facial plastic surgery in the Department of Otolaryngology. He is an internationally known lecturer to many continuing medical education societies and universities in the United States, Mexico, and Britain.

Dr. Ellis has published thirty articles in peer-reviewed journals on facial plastic surgery, and written twelve chapters in books on facial plastic surgery. He is an author of *About Face—A Consumer's Guide to Facial Cosmetic Surgery in Canada* (Macmillan Canada, 1992). He is also coauthor of *Your Complete Guide to Nose Reshaping* (Addicus Books, 2007).

Dr. Ellis's honors include being the founding president of the Canadian Academy of Facial Plastic Surgery, and past president of the Canadian Society of Otolaryngology—Head and Neck Surgery. He has been elected to the board of the American Academy of Facial Plastic and Reconstructive Surgery as the Canadian vice president and again as director-at-large.

Dr. Ellis is a member of the Canadian Academy of Facial Plastic Surgery, the American Academy of Facial Plastic and Reconstructive Surgery, the Canadian Society of Otolaryngology—Head and Neck Surgery, the American Academy of Cosmetic Surgery, the Canadian Medical Association, and the Ontario Medical Association. He is president of the Canadian Academy of Facial Plastic and Reconstructive Surgery and is the Canadian delegate to the International Federation of Facial Plastic Surgical Societies (IFFPSS).

For more information about Dr. Ellis and the procedures he performs, visit his Web site: **www.artoffacialsurgery.com.**

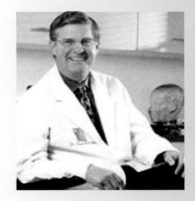

"With the technology available today, facial cosmetic procedures of all types can be performed safely and with results that look very natural."

—David Ellis, M.D.

Consumer Health Titles
from Addicus Books

Visit our online catalog at www.AddicusBooks.com

After Mastectomy—Healing Physically and Emotionally	$14.95
Body Contouring after Weight Loss	$21.95
Cancers of the Mouth and Throat A Patient's Guide to Treatment	$14.95
Cataracts: A Patient's Guide to Treatment	$14.95
The Clarins Concept	$19.95
Colon & Rectal Cancer—A Patient's Guide to Treatment	$14.95
Coping with Psoriasis—A Patient's Guide to Treatment	$14.95
Coronary Heart Disease—A Guide to Diagnosis and Treatment	$15.95
Countdown to Baby	$14.95
Elder Care Made Easier	$16.95
Exercising Through Your Pregnancy	$17.95
The Fertility Handbook—A Guide to Getting Pregnant	$14.95
The Healing Touch—Keeping the Doctor/Patient Relationship Alive Under Managed Care	$9.95
LASIK—A Guide to Laser Vision Correction	$14.95
Living with P.C.O.S.—Polycystic Ovarian Syndrome	$14.95
Look Out Cancer Here I Come	$19.95
Lung Cancer—A Guide to Treatment & Diagnosis	$14.95
The Macular Degeneration Source Book	$14.95
The New Fibromyalgia Remedy	$16.95
The Non-Surgical Facelift Book A Guide to Facial Rejuvenation Procedures	$14.95

Overcoming Metabolic Syndrome	$14.95
Overcoming Postpartum Depression and Anxiety	$14.95
A Patient's Guide to Dental Implants	$14.95
Prescription Drug Addiction—The Hidden Epidemic	$15.95
Prostate Cancer—A Patient's Guide to Treatment	$14.95
Simple Changes: The Boomer's Guide to a Healthier, Happier Life	$9.95
A Simple Guide to Thyroid Disorders	$14.95
Straight Talk About Breast Cancer From Diagnosis to Recovery	$14.95
The Stroke Recovery Book A Guide for Patients and Families	$14.95
The Surgery Handbook—A Guide to Understanding Your Operation	$14.95
Understanding Lumpectomy A Treatment Guide for Breast Cancer	$14.95
Understanding Parkinson's Disease A Self-Help Guide	$14.95
Understanding Peyronie's Disease	$16.95
Understanding Your Living Will	$12.95
Your Complete Guide to Breast Augmentation & Body Contouring	$21.95
Your Complete Guide to Breast Reduction & Breast Lifts	$21.95
Your Complete Guide to Facial Cosmetic Surgery	$19.95
Your Complete Guide to Facial Rejuvenation	$21.95
Your Complete Guide to Nose Reshaping	$21.95

Order online at: www.addicusbooks.com or Toll Free: 800-342-2873.

Organizations, associations, corporations, hospitals, and other groups may qualify for special discounts when ordering more than 24 copies. For more information, please contact the Special Sales Department at Addicus Books. Phone (402) 330-7493.
Email: info@AddicusBooks.com